HOPE
An Inspiring A - Z Guide for Cancer Patients, Survivors and Caregivers

D1528415

HOPE

An Inspiring A - Z Guide for Cancer Patients, Survivors and Caregivers

Patti McGee
Author & Survivor

Book and cover design by Deborah Kress Smith
Photos by Jude Hefferon

ISBN: 978-0-615-46510-4

Publisher: Patti McGee

Author: Patti McGee

Email: pmcgee2@twcny.rr.com

My Dedication

As a breast cancer survivor, I am always looking for ways to educate and assist cancer patients, survivors and their caregivers to help make their journey through cancer easier. Although no two patients' treatments are exactly the same, having to endure treatment and follow-up appointments for years, we all go through similar concerns about our disease.

I dedicate this book to my son Dylan, the most precious gift I ever received in my life; my parents, Karen and "Fibber;" my siblings, Kelly, Colleen, Shawn and Tim, who all stood by me through my treatment and continuing journey with cancer.

To my special friends Lisa Thomas, Sandra Miller, and Penny Poling who have all been a tremendous support to each other and me through our journey and given unselfishly to newly diagnosed cancer patients. Your true friendship is always cherished.

To my medical team, especially Karen Litwak and Mickey Moore, who are the most dedicated healthcare professionals in Central New York.

I would like to thank the following individuals who have all helped me bring my book from a dream to reality: life coach, Teresa Huggins, my editors MaryAnne Buteux, Mike Jaquays and CeCe Flyzik and my cousin Deb Smith for helping me design the cover and the book style.

Lastly, I would like to thank all the survivors and caregivers who have contributed their stories. Through your stories, we can assist other newly diagnosed patients through their journeys and give them the courage to continue to fight this disease. Without your contributions, this book would still be a dream.

Thank you and God Bless.

Patricia A. McGee
April 2011

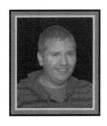

Special Dedication

I dedicate this page to my son Dylan. No words can express the gratitude I have towards you for your strength and resilience since my cancer diagnosis in 2002. I can only say thank you for your kind words when I was feeling down; thank you for the laughter when I felt no hope; and thank you for your love when I felt defeated.

At the age of 9, as I lay there sick after each treatment, you were there to wipe my face with a warm washcloth and empty my vomit bucket. When I felt ugly from radiation tattoo markers and being bald from losing my hair you would remind me that beauty is only skin deep; that it is what is on the inside of a person that truly matters as I had told you so many times.

I have watched you grow over the years from a child into a handsome young man and I want to say thank you for your continued support during the rollercoaster ride this cancer journey has taken us on. I am very proud to have you as my son; your smile lights up a room, your humor fills a room with laughter and your kindness opens so many hearts.

You and so many other children experience so much in watching a loved one go through their cancer journey, but at the end of the day you become stronger, wiser and learn what unconditional love truly means.

I look forward to spending many more years watching you grow and pursue your dreams. Remember that you are only limited by your imagination and you can do anything you put your mind to. I encourage you to dream big and live life to its fullest.

Love,

Mom

Foreword

In December of 2002, I found myself sitting across from my surgeon and hearing him say those three little but powerful words "You have Cancer." Since that day, my life has changed for the better, although at times it didn't seem like it.

As with all cancer patients, I started with the tests of blood work and scans to see if the cancer had spread anywhere else in my body and I remember I had to wait until December 26, 2002 to receive the results. It was one of the most trying times of my life. I was so distraught that Christmas that year is a blur. Being a single mother, I didn't have the strength to decorate the Christmas tree. I remember my son Dylan telling me that it was okay that we didn't finish decorating the tree as long as we were together. He is wise beyond his years. Then the day after Christmas came and my surgeon called and gave me the good news that the cancer had not spread, but they couldn't get a clear margin so we had to schedule another lumpectomy.

A partial mastectomy and removal of 21 lymph nodes brought about chemotherapy and radiation. That journey will have to be told in another book. The next seven years have been filled with triumphs and tribulations between treatments, learning who the "New Me" was and is and my relationship with my family and co-workers.

My main focus in writing this book is to help guide and give inspiration to newly diagnosed patients, survivors and their supporters by providing them with some basic and simple information they can understand and refer back to throughout their journey. I have included several survivor stories to help provide you with inspiration and to let you know you are not alone in this journey.

I hope you find this book useful and inspiring.

Table of Contents

NOTES FROM THE ONCOLOGY OFFICE

Take A Proactive Approach
Karen Litwak, ANP
SUNY UPSTATE
Regional Oncology Office
Oneida, NY

I am a health care provider in a busy oncology office where cancer patients are seen daily. Patients handle the diagnosis of cancer differently. Some want to know everything about their disease and the treatment by researching and using the Internet. Then there are those who say, "Just tell me what treatment to take but don't give me much information." It is beneficial if the patient and their family take a proactive approach to the diagnosis and treatment options.

What does proactive mean? Every patient should have a journal or notebook that includes dates, symptoms, pathology, surgeries, blood work and x-ray testing done with the results. Notations should also include doctor visits, medication list, allergies, and treatments. Everyone should learn the basic information about their diagnosis, including stage, where the disease is and their treatment options. Many patients feel the doctor should decide the treatment plan. Patients who are involved with the decisions planning their treatment actually tolerate treatments better and listen to our recommendations about managing side effects. Each patient should have a list of questions they have compiled since their last visit. It is difficult for anyone to remember every issue they want to discuss at their doctor's visit.   It is also important to bring someone with you to your appointments. Another person will pick up different information from a discussion. It will be easier when you try to recall what the doctor says if you can discuss it with another family member who heard the same discussion.

All this information is not easy to understand or absorb when you are coping with a new cancer diagnosis. With a second opinion, another doctor may agree with the diagnosis and recommend the same treatments. However, many times the patient and the family are more receptive to the discussion and able to ask questions at a second opinion appointment.

Many patients will ask "When am I considered a survivor?" The American Cancer Society defines the cancer patient as a survivor from the day of diagnosis. The American Cancer Society is a free reliable resource for you and your family.

Your caregiver is a very important part of your journey with cancer. Patients need to involve their caregiver in their decisions and difficulties with treatments. Your caregiver loves you very much and may feel very helpless.

It is most important that you do not sit home if you are ill. Be sure you call your physician. Also do not hesitate to call if you have any questions. Every physician has coverage 24 hours per day. There are many supportive drugs and advice your provider can offer. They cannot help if they do not know you are ill. Everyone tolerates treatments differently.

Always remember there are new treatments and drugs being developed. Looking back on the developments related to cancer care in the past 15 years, I realize how far we have come. I feel that with further research and more new drugs, there will be a cure for cancer.

Side note from the Author:

Karen is a very dedicated and professional Nurse Practitioner. In 2003 and 2004, we joined together in conjunction with the American Cancer Society to offer two support groups and start a Relay For Life. She has been very instrumental in getting guest speakers and sponsorships for our I Can Cope series and monthly support group meetings. She works diligently to provide the patients with the best possible treatment available to them and reaches out when they are in need. Karen has helped bring over one million dollars to the Oneida area through the American Cancer Society's Relay For Life to provide programs such as the Look Good Feel Better Program, a monthly support group, the I Can Cope series and to provide funding for mileage for those in need to get to their treatments.

Karen has assisted me through some of the darkest moments in my life and has always been there as a nurse practitioner, confidant and friend. I dedicate this page to her for her selflessness and many hours of dedication to her patients and community.

Notes from the Doctor's Office

Life's Changing Moments
By Michele "Mickey" Moore, ANP-C
Oneida OBGYN Group
Oneida, NY

"Connie, give me your hand." "Can you feel this?" At that point in time everything changes for Connie, it's inevitable that at that exact moment life will be very different for her. It doesn't matter if her lump is cancerous or benign; she will never be quite the same, and she can't be. She has now experienced every emotion possible in one flash moment. If her diagnosis is cancer she will face the most difficult, emotional time of her life. I can assure you, however, for a fact, it is also a beginning. After 30 years in women's health, I have learned that there is no easy way to say, "I think this may be cancerous."

Let me share with you some thoughts and emotions that are part of me and most likely all healthcare providers, at the prospect of a suspected cancer for one of our patients. I first think about who this person is and how they may handle this news. I then, usually, sit down and say, "We need to do further testing." I try very hard to not say "cancer," at least at first. The reason for this is I will lose the person and my words will not be heard. I can often see the fear in her eyes. I also feel overwhelmed with emotions. I can tell you, though, that almost instantly - every time - I feel love from her, and love for her family, her friends and herself. Let me tell you at that point, this woman's life has flashed before her eyes; she suddenly is much more worried about how to tell her loved ones the news.

Secondly, I explain the importance of understanding and following through with testing and appointments. This can be especially difficult for some people because of denial. Denial can persuade some to say, "I can't possibly do that tomorrow" or "I can't do that right now." If your healthcare provider recommends you do something, try very hard to find a way to do it. Remember that putting off a test or procedure can cause serious consequences. When you postpone an appointment, you postpone recovery.

Be informed, be your own advocate, ask questions and most importantly listen to the answers. Repeat information back to your provider to make sure you understand, take someone with you, and write things down; it helps to retain as much as possible. You will hear things differently. It can be vital to have someone else be your ears. No question is stupid and your question may very well help someone else. I will remember your questions and build on them when I am sitting with someone in a similar situation.

Don't be afraid to be strong willed. Be a consumer of your own healthcare. Shop, investigate, consider and follow through. Just don't postpone. Ask, "Why?" "What will that do?" "How will that affect me?" Read from a prepared list of questions and make sure you plan, construct and build your future. Set realistic goals, start with short term goals and move forward. Smile. Do things that make you happy, surround yourself with others who are supportive yet not overly protective. You will need room to grow and time for yourself. Your life will change and what direction it takes depends on you. In my years of caring for women, I have seen how a cancer diagnosis creates much stronger souls, stronger relationships and stronger personalities.

The most important advice I can leave you with is that you need to hug your family, hug your friends, even yourself, but don't forget to hug your healthcare provider. They love you too.

> **Side note from the Author:**
>
> In March 2010, Mickey Moore was the recipient of the Status of Women Award by the Zonta Club of Oneida for her dedication to improving and maintaining a quality of life for women and their families through health, education and safety (Oneida Daily Dispatch, March 2010).
>
> I first met Mickey as my OBGYN when I was having some problems after my cancer treatments were over and she told me she would be honored to have me as a patient. She is a very sincere, dedicated and caring nurse practitioner. I dedicate this page to her for all she does for her patients to improve their quality of life through mind, body and spirit. There are not many doctors or nurses who give their phone numbers out to their patients and tell them to call any time, day or night, if they have a concern or question, but Mickey is one of them and she is sincere about it. Mickey has been an inspiration and true friend to me throughout my cancer journey.

Message from a Cosmetologist

A Temporary Time in Your Life
Kelly McGee, Owner
Hair Razors Hair Salon
Whitesboro, NY

I graduated in June 1980 from the cosmetology program at the Oneida Herkimer Madison B.O.C.E.S. I have always known that I wanted to work as a hair stylist and have been fortunate to own my own business for several years. Over the years I have taught cosmetology at B.O.C.E.S, worked as an instructor for Redkin and volunteered for the American Cancer Society's Look Good Feel Better program.

Through the Look Good Feel Better program, as a stylist, I have had to shave several women's heads due to losing their hair from chemotherapy. I have had to go through this experience many times and the one thought that I have is that you have to keep thinking "This is a temporary time in my life". Everyone deals with it differently. As a support person, you have to let them feel what they feel and just listen to how they express it! Some of my clients look at it as a time to experiment and buy a wig in red, blonde or brunette. Others want one that matches their natural hair as close as possible. Family can influence this decision greatly, so be careful what your reaction is and remember to be supportive no matter what. It is my experience that if the side effects weren't so physically visible some people would have an easier emotional time. It is like watching a slow train wreck. You avoid one side effect only to get two others! I probably had shaved 10 clients' heads but the one I remember most was when I had to shave my sister's head.

I remember like it was yesterday. It was March 2003, a cold and snowy Sunday when she called me saying she couldn't stand it anymore! She had been in the shower and clumps of hair were falling out all over. I hopped in my truck and drove to her house. I cried all the way there and all the way home but not while I was there! What was good was that my sister was never very vain to begin with so she didn't miss her hair as much as I did. Once it started to come in, she grew it out for Locks for Love. You need 12" to send to them. I bet if you asked her she would say that that was harder than shaving it! Ironic isn't it?

If you know you are going to lose your hair from chemotherapy, women who take a proactive approach and start out by cutting it shorter prior to losing it have an easier time when it comes time to shave it.

Side note from the Author:

Kelly is my sister and the bond that we formed during my treatment is very special to me. We shared a lot of laughter on that day she shaved my head, although it was tough for both of us and neither of us wanted to cry in front of the other. Kelly has always been very good at reaching out in time of need. When I was going through a very rough stretch due to side effects of some medications, she would always be there asking the right questions and also giving me my space to learn and grow. I just want to say thank you for all you do to help others through their journey and for being there for me when I need it most.

A Message from Camp Good Days and Special Times

A Time for Reflection
Wendy Mervis, Executive Director
Mendon, NY

Camp Good Days and Special Times began over 30 years ago as a summer camp for children with cancer. Camp Good Days remains dedicated to improving the quality of life for children and families whose lives have been touched by cancer and other life threatening challenges, through residential camping experiences held at their own, beautiful recreational facility on Keuka Lake. They also offer year-round recreational and support activities and events held across Upstate New York in Rochester, Buffalo, Syracuse, and the Southern Tier Region, for families who are facing life's toughest challenges.

While nothing at Camp Good Days will find a cure for cancer or other life threatening challenges, everything is done in an effort to create some good days and special times for the children and families served. Camp Good Days is a celebration of life, with those who have learned to appreciate it the most ... a place where courage knows no boundaries.

Over the past 30 years the camp has expanded to offer various programs for siblings, children and adults who have a family member with cancer. One of our most popular adult programs is our Women's Oncology Weekends. Women from all over the country who have been diagnosed with any type of cancer come to camp to be with others who are going through or have gone through the same situation and seek hope for the future.

I think one of the most meaningful activities that we have at our Women's Oncology Program at Camp Good Days is our closing ceremony in the outdoor chapel. It is a time of reflection, closure, and peace. By coming together one last time, everyone is able to think about all that has happened over the weekend. The outdoor chapel, set in the trees and by the creek, is a truly peaceful place. Taking an hour to think and to share prayer is a truly comforting experience. The most prolific part of the closing ceremony is the rock that one can choose to leave behind. Each person is given a rock from the creek that has been painted white. Each person can write what they want on the rock. Whether it is the name of someone in your family you are thinking of, yourself, or a friend that you miss or is going through a hard time, it is up to each person what they choose to write. Then you can place the rock under the large wooden cross or Star of David that are set in the ground. These rocks will always be there, unmoved. There are hundreds of rocks that have accumulated through the years, and the pile gets higher. It symbolizes that everyone who has passed through camp has left a piece of themselves there and it will remain.

Many of the women leave camp with many new friends and a kindred spirit. For more information on Camp Good Days and Special Times please visit our website at www.campgooddays.org.

Message from a Massage Therapist

Cancer and Massage Therapy
By Barb Villanti, LMT; PT

Years ago, a myth in massage therapy existed that massage was an absolute contraindication for the cancer population, probably out of fear that increasing circulation could cause the spread of cancer. This generalization caused therapists to avoid massage all together for those that had cancer. But in recent years, this had been challenged and closely examined. The assumption that massage would increase circulation that could cause cancer cells to spread was not accurate. If this were the case, physicians would have limited one's exercise for fear this would increase blood and lymph flow, thereby causing cancer cells to spread.

Massage therapy has been a growing trend. Once thought a luxury, it is now part of one's healthcare. While there are many reasons people receive a massage, medical massage is expanding. According to the American Massage Therapy Association, 48 million adult Americans (22%) had a massage at least once between July 2008 and July 2009. Thirty two percent of those had a massage for medical or health reasons. The medical community is embracing and discussing the use of massage therapy with their patients as an integral part of their health and well being. Massage has been incorporated into many medical oncology centers/hospitals and hospice programs for the recovery process of someone going through cancer and its treatment.

Once you have been diagnosed with cancer and then go through the treatment, patients are focused on one thing ... eradicating the cancer. Anything else can be dealt with at a later time. That goes for any side effects from the cancer and its treatment. Oncology massage can help to restore your body and spirit. By integrating massage into your treatment you can address your symptoms. Patients can experience a variety of symptoms during and after their cancer treatment. Such symptoms patients can feel are, but not limited to, pain, nausea, fatigue, depression, stress/anxiety, swelling/lymphedema, and tightness/stiffness from scar adhesions and a disconnection from their bodies.

A three year study at Memorial Sloan Kettering Cancer Center consisting of 1290 patients has shown that massage eases the side effects of pain, nausea, fatigue and depression, at least in the short term. Compared with drug therapies for these symptoms, massage is as effective, cheaper, less invasive, more comforting and free of further side effects. Research continues to show the benefits of massage but more studies need to be done. Researchers caution that while massage may offer some immediate relief for patients with cancer, effects do not last over time.

The benefits of massage:

Relaxation. When your body is stressed your immune system is less able to fight off disease. Touch can release chemicals like endorphins in the body to help us relax, improve circulation, reduce muscle spasms, and strengthen our immune system.

Pain reduction. Pain is one of the most common symptoms of cancer patients and is a quality of life issue. Consequences of pain include isolation, fatigue, depression, and more visits to the doctor's office. Massage restores pleasurable touch.

Body Awareness. Due to traditional treatment (surgery, radiation and chemotherapy), treatment can affect one's body image. Massage can create body awareness and increase mind body connection.

Reduction of scar tissue. Scarring is unavoidable due to surgery and radiation. Scarring is not only a cosmetic issue but can also cause pain, tightness and possibly a collection of fluid in an area due to scar tissue adhesions. A therapist can perform techniques that can realign the fibers and reduce the adhesions.

Reduction of swelling. Are you at risk for lymphedema? Lymphedema is a high protein fluid in the tissues causing swelling in the affected arm and the adjacent quadrant. Oncology massage therapy integrates safety protocols especially if lymph nodes have been compromised. If you have swelling in your arm or adjacent quadrant after breast cancer treatment you need to contact your doctor. There can be various reasons you can have swelling: post surgical, blood clot or lymphedema. You need to seek out a certified lymphedema therapist to provide you with the proper massage treatment of manual lymphatic drainage.

Your massage therapist should have a thorough knowledge of cancer and its treatment, the correct amount of pressure to use, what areas to avoid and potential side effects. Prior to attending your massage session, discuss massage with your doctor first, in cases of any precautions or contraindications such as the following: blood clots, taking blood thinning or anticoagulant medication, low platelet counts, skin fragility after radiation, infections, bone metastasis, congestive heart failure.

Aa - Attitude

ဆာ

Keeping a positive attitude from the day of diagnosis will help you to be strong before, during and after treatment. Make positive affirmations part of your daily routine. Research shows that patients have a higher success rate of survival if they keep a positive attitude throughout their diagnosis and treatment. Join a support group and talk about your diagnosis to help you focus on the positive aspects of your treatment. Surrounding yourself with positive people will give you the support you need to make it through your treatments.

Have an Attitude of Gratitude that you are alive.

Stronger Than Before
Sandra Miller
Verona, NY

It all started just before Christmas of 2002. I felt a lump under my left breast and knew that wasn't right so I called my OBGYN. She saw me instantly and decided it must be removed and biopsied. When I returned to the doctor's office for my follow up appointment with my mother and young son, I was given the news that I had breast cancer. All of a sudden I had all these thoughts going through my mind, "Is this a good kind of cancer or a bad kind?" What did I know about having cancer? No one in my family or any of my friends have cancer, so why me? The doctor told me there is no "good" kind of cancer.

At the time of my diagnosis I wasn't too freaked out by the thought of having cancer because people deal with this every day, right? I could too. Someone told me "You need to give up one year of your life to live 30 more." I could do this. So I took off 11 months at my job in a receiving department to get completely healed. I loved everyone I worked with and my job. During the 11 months, I stayed home to recuperate from surgery, chemotherapy and radiation. I was able to spend time with my husband Eric, 2-year-old son Dustin and my 5-year-old daughter Taylor, who was in kindergarten. I rested when my children napped and things were going good.

In January 2004, I was back at work and things were looking up. I was going to the oncologist every three months and my next appointment was approaching. I went for my recheck and that is when I was told that my cancer had returned. My first thought was how that could be after all I had been through. My doctor explained to me how the cancer cells find weak spots in the body and grow. I asked her what that means and she told me "We are going to be very good friends."   I liked having friends and all but I had a feeling she wasn't going to be inviting me for coffee. Sure enough, it wasn't coffee she was going to be serving; it was going to be a cocktail of chemotherapy.

I had a port put in to make administering the chemotherapy easier and I definitely would recommend it to anyone having chemotherapy; it is much easier on the veins. I was able to continue working and I got involved with our local Relay For Life and support groups. Work was my escape from cancer and the support groups and Relay helped me to stay positive.

   Over the next couple years my cancer continued to spread even during treatment so I had to quit my job in May 2005. Although at times it was hard, thinking about the alternative was not an option. Some time went by and things were looking good; my family and I were able to spend some time together and camp. There is nothing like family and friends to help you through your disease. Through our local support group I was invited to attend Camp Good Days and Special Times Women's Oncology weekend and was able to talk to other women who were going through a similar diagnosis. I enjoyed Camp Good Days so much that my children now attend each year. One thing that is different from other survivors and me is that most survivors fear that their cancer will return, but with me having cancer throughout my body I don't worry about when it will return.

   In May 2007 I was having headaches. I self-diagnosed myself with migraines but I found out that the breast cancer had metastasized to my brain and I had to have another surgery. Over the past few years, I was able to stay positive with each recurrence but this time it really bothered me! I wanted this to be it. I mean, enough is enough already. This wasn't my choice, but I knew God had his own plan for me and dying isn't it. I have to admit sometimes it was hard, but while I was recuperating from the brain surgery a friend of mine called Bill Bryant, a minister, to come talk to me in the hospital. He made me realize that life was worth fighting for and to keep a positive attitude for each day that I was alive. Over the past few years I have had a few small tumors return and I go in for gamma knife surgery which is an in and out procedure so I am back home with my family that day.

With all the new metastasis', my chemotherapies have changed from IVs to oral medications. I was given xeloda, tykerb and a handful of others but it is the perfect cocktail to keep cancer away. I was cruising along, until May of 2009 when I was feeling tired and just couldn't stay awake. I had taken my son to school and the next thing I remember was my husband asking me, "Why are you sitting in the car and why are you parked in the bushes?" I didn't recall the drive home. My husband loaded me in the car and we were off to the ER. Days later the diagnosis came in and my adrenal glands were not producing the necessary hormones so they gave me some more pills to take. I felt like I was in an episode of the TV show "House."

I wasn't home a couple days before we had our annual Relay For Life in June 2009 and with the medication for my adrenal glands I was able to stay awake the whole 16 hours through the night. It was so inspiring. I remember other survivors telling me that I am their inspiration. Months went on and once again I was told that the cancer was worse in my liver. I should have given the cancer a name had I known it was going to be part of my family.

Now what? A different chemotherapy? Will I lose my hair (this is an important question unless you are already bald) or will I get sick? My doctor is always honest with me and I feel this is very important. You need to have a good relationship with your doctor.

Try not to dwell on your sorrows; embrace them, and turn them into something good whenever you can. Know who your support system is and use them.

I am fortunate to have a wonderful family and strong faith in God to help me through the good and bad times. I know my cancer will never be completely gone but with new research and medications I am proof that research works. I often feel really good and don't worry about things. I take it one day at a time and let the doctors do the worrying. I am hopeful that someday there will be a cure.

Side note from the Author

At the time of publication my friend and inspiration Sandra Miller passed away due to breast cancer. Over the past eight years Sandra, throughout her battle, was such an inspiration to many survivors. She overcame so many metastases throughout her body and always kept a positive attitude. A few years ago in June, she was hospitalized due to her adrenal glands shutting down and when she was released a couple days before our local Relay For Life, Sandra walked and stayed awake the whole 16 hours of the Relay. Her love for life and her family was so inspiring. Sandra was a good friend, mother, wife, daughter and aunt to many. Although she will be missed dearly, her legacy through her fight and journey with cancer will live on through the Oneida Area for years to come.

Bb - Breathe and Believe

☙ ❧

Learn to breathe to help keep that positive attitude and clear your mind of any negative thoughts. Learning to breathe will help you to relax in any stressful situation you find yourself in. As a massage therapist, when I ask my clients to take a deep breath they tend to breathe in through their mouth and tighten their abdominal muscles when in reality they should be breathing in through their nose, extending their abdomen and then exhaling out through their mouth. While breathing you should be able to feel your lungs fill with air, feel it move through your body, down your legs to your toes and down your arms to your fingertips.

A breathing technique that I have found to work is to sit up straight on the floor or in a chair; close your eyes and breathe in through your nose filling your lungs, chest and abdomen with air; at the same time, bring your arms from your side, up over your head and then exhale slowly through your mouth and lower your arms back to your side. Repeat ten to twelve times. Think of it as "smelling the flowers and then blowing out birthday candles."

Controlled breathing can be a form of meditation; it helps you to focus on your body and mind and remove any of the little voices in your head that might be giving you negative thoughts or an overactive mind. I have talked with several caregivers and one of the biggest complaints of the cancer survivor is the inability to sleep after treatment is over because we start wondering if we really are cancer free, how do we know if the treatment worked, and is there something else I should be doing to prevent the cancer from coming back. These are normal thoughts and will diminish with time. There are some medication prescriptions your healthcare provider can give you but make sure you talk to them first before taking anything.

Seeing the Signs - Faith vs. Religion vs. Relationships
By Barry Depot
Utica, NY

There once was a story about a faithful God follower. She goes to Heaven and at the pearly gates she proceeds to ask why God hadn't saved her from the flood? Saint Peter asks her "When the water was at the front steps of your house - why didn't you go with the firefighters and the policemen?" The faithful woman said "I figured God would save me." So Saint Peter asks, "When the water was up to your windows, do you remember that guy with the boat?" "Yes, of course," the faithful follower says. "But you stayed – why?" "Because I had faith the good Lord would save me." "And when the water was at roof level – and you waved off the helicopter – what were you thinking then?" "That God would somehow come and save me!" So Saint Peter says to his faithful servant, "Well then, who do you think sent the firemen and police, the boat and the helicopter?"

Sometimes we just fail to see the signs - don't we?

My story is fairly simple: I was born and raised to be a faithful Catholic. Our family was devout - rarely did we miss a week of Mass, even if on vacation. When I went to college, as many kids do, I drifted away from the church. Overall I was a pretty good guy - I married a Jewish girl, my high-school sweetheart, and we raised two "cashews" (Catholic-Jews). But our new family together wasn't connected to a church let alone to a religion. Three of my five siblings have converted to the Baptist faith over the years. The few times that I would visit them I would typically attend their church services and while I personally got a lot out of their churches by getting that hair raising, goose pimply, and unexplained welling in the eyes reaction - I failed to act on those signs and lead my family towards something greater.

After all, life, the kids, the jobs, the community involvement, the coaching, the cancer ... well, it all just kind of got in the way. After all, I couldn't imagine taking another hour from my precious week - how was I really going to squeeze an hour or two for God with an already full and stressful life? There needed to be time made for God, but where were the signs?

My story complicates: In 1997, at the ripe old age of 30, I was diagnosed with chronic lymphocytic leukemia (CLL). Sure, I had heard of leukemia but I had no idea what CLL was, let alone that it was a form of "a cancer of the blood." Immediately after my diagnosis, I had never really felt that alone in my entire life - like I was the only one that I knew that had cancer. Was this a sign I was looking for? Was I even looking for a sign? And if so, what kind of sign was this? For most of us getting a sign like this just doesn't feel good at all. And it didn't.

Prior to being diagnosed with cancer, I had a pretty good idea of who I was but once diagnosed, it both refined me and defined me. It put my entire life in focus on a possible timeline that was not acceptable to me and my family. In fact, if I had listened to the first booklet of information I read about CLL, I would not be typing this story at all. But not seeing my children graduate from high school was not an option to me. Now, in 2010, with one son already graduated from high school - and with one son to graduate in 2012 - I look forward to college graduations, weddings and grand children - followed by a wonderful lengthy retirement with my wife of over 22 years.

Fortunately, I've never felt like a victim to cancer. As strange as this may sound, I've felt that the cancer has been a blessing from the very beginning. I've been able to address many programs sponsored by the American Cancer Society as one of their 2010 Heroes of Hope and tell them that cancer has truly been an incredible gift from God. Even though I went from patient to survivor after my first treatment - when I had one of those "one in a thousand reactions" - the "Barney the purple dinosaur" face, the falling blood pressure, the headache, the flu-like symptoms - and I lived through it all, only to be treated again the next day - that's when I became a survivor. That was back in April of 1999. I was so thankful to survive my first day of treatment. I realized then how much God needed to be part of my life - and I in His.

The story continues: Some years later, I was perplexed about a busy week ahead. I took a Monday off of work to golf with my brother and I knew the shortened week was going to be hectic. I worked Tuesday and that night I got a call from a soccer coach buddy of mine that I hadn't talked to in months. It was 9:00 pm and though I was ready for bed, my friend invited himself over to my house to show me a car on the Internet that he was going to buy. We visited for about an hour and we had a few good laughs. As we discussed getting together again and looking at possible dates, he mentioned he was going that week to a Bible study so I asked if I could go with him and he said "Yes; I'm sure." So my religious journey was seemingly back on some sort of track. But the most amazing thing about our "happenstance" meeting in this story was the fact that during my brother's four hour trip home that day, he had prayed that God would bring someone into my life and bring the fire in my belly about God as I had had with my kids' baseball and their soccer. This was a big sign - as big as ever in my life. So Bible study began in earnest that week.

Proudly, some seven years later, I am very happy to say that I haven't missed more than a handful of Bible studies (whether on a Thursday, Wednesday, Monday, or Tuesday since we've hopped around a bit given everyone's busy morning schedules). In fact, while I was away from home in 2008 for several months having a bone marrow transplant (BMT) at the Mayo Clinic in Rochester, MN, our group still met and I participated via video using the Internet and Skype. We've had people drop in and out of our little group but what I've gotten most out of Bible study is through the growing relationship with God, and the camaraderie of a few lost souls I have an appreciation that God can work in very mysterious ways. We sometimes question, and often wonder why the answers are not always self evident. Sometimes there is no "in your face" sign.

Sometimes the answers may never seem to come - at least not to our satisfaction and understanding. Sometimes we still miss the signs - especially if we're not looking for them.

Through all the potential pain and this incredible journey, I have also come to learn that which doesn't kill you makes you stronger starting with my diagnosis of CLL in 1997 - it hasn't killed me yet. The chemotherapy in 1999, 2003, 2005, 2007 and 2008 - made me feel tired, energized, as well as different, but it did not kill me. The fungal infection in 2006 that hospitalized me for ten days - it came darn close to killing me, but it didn't. The two transplants - my own stem-cells in 2003 and again, a Matched Unrelated Donor (MUD) BMT in 2008 - they tried to kill me, but didn't. The "lymphocyte-storm" that overwhelmed my lungs in 2009 - put me on a ventilator, shut down my lungs, then my kidneys and then my liver - that was the closest one yet, but it did not kill me. And now in 2010, as I write this from the 6th floor of my local hospital with pneumonia - it has not even come close to killing me - and in fact, I laugh at this feeble attempt.

So, through all of this refining, I have come to love all people and "their" story. Who they are, why they are, where they've been, where they are going, and how I somehow might fit in - if at all. Each and every interaction is sweeter, more interesting and more important than ever. So where's the sign? How about this - if I have been through all of this, and survived to talk and write about it, then why not you? What is so special about me and my story? Aren't you as special to God as I am? There is no doubt in my military mind.

And I have to tell you, since the ventilator incident in 2009, everything in life is more colorful, more noticeable and more vibrant - like I'm at a new level of consciousness. And when someone is having a bad day, or even if things aren't going well for me, all I have to say or think is, "Well, it is better than being on the ventilator," or, "It is better than the alternative," and people just simply smile, and they typically turn their head to the one side - nod in agreement, and say "You know, you are right - what am I complaining about?" And with those simple words, it seems to diffuse most situations and just make things better.

I have many other "God stories" but I felt like this one might reach out to people who are looking for a sign. While my life was amazing prior to cancer - I mean, I already had a wonderful wife, two adoring kids, a successful career, a beautiful home - but I was truly missing something. I had a hole in my heart that yearned to be filled. Thankfully, through the perseverance of my brother and my long lost soccer friend I finally began to see the many signs He was posting for me up and down my street telling me "you need God in your life." It wasn't until then I finally climbed up the ladder to the helicopter - and here's the golden nugget - it is not enough for you see the sign, but you need to act on the sign in order to gain something from it.

Because of this very personal act - as if God was in my living room that night and as my relationship with God has blossomed - my faith has never been greater. So in order to survive cancer you must also have faith in a higher power and remember that no matter what, we all must realize a couple of things. Number one: We're just not in charge. Number two: We are not going to get out of this thing called "life" alive. Number three: What is most important is what we do with that time between now (life) and then (not alive). Number four: That by these pages, by this book, by our treatments, by our trials and tribulation, and by our relationships, we're all in this together. And last, but certainly not least, number five: Never take cancer too serious - it might kill you! I've embraced my sense of humor and I encourage others to find humor in all the crazy stuff that happens to us as cancer survivors and caregivers. It is helpful and extremely important that while cancer is serious stuff - you must learn to laugh often and things will go much better than expected!

Bottom line, my faith and the comfort from God's gift of grace has truly filled that void in my heart. It has carried me and my family through very difficult and scary times with my disease, the treatments, and the near-death experiences. I am certain that God wanted us together here today - for me to write this story - and for you to hear it right here, and right now. So here is your sign. Don't let the helicopter leave you behind. How will you act on it? How will you let God save you? To me that is as personal as His visit to me in my living room to where you are now. Seek the sign. See the sign. Act on the sign. We plan on seeing each and every one of you up in Heaven!

Cc - Caregiver

ಐಓಚ

The caregiver(s) will be the most important individuals or people in your life. They will be there for you and you need to let them know how you are feeling so they can help you. Be open and honest with them so they know how to assist you through your treatment process and journey.

When you are first diagnosed, do not be surprised that some individuals you thought you could count on are not there for you and the ones you thought wouldn't be there to help you will be by your side throughout the whole journey. You will meet and form what we survivors call our "new family" of friends. My circle of friends has completely changed over the past 7 years.

One very important thing to remember is to let people help you. If you have someone that wants to make dinner for you and your family accept the help. Everyone around you will want to help you in different ways which will help them to accept your diagnosis.

Celebrate each new day! Julie Hanna
(2007 Lessons for Life Calendar)

I Am Here For You
Jerry Compoli
Oneida, NY

On Wednesday, March 31, 2004 I remember going with my wife Jan for her biopsy appointment. I felt this would all be routine and nothing would be wrong. My wife Jan was very sick after her hospital visit from the anesthesia. She rested that afternoon, and was fine the next morning.

On Wednesday, April 7, 2004 at 4:30 pm, I went with my wife to see her surgeon for results of the biopsy. I felt I needed to go with her, although I felt there really would be nothing wrong. She was called in and I waited in the reception area. The doctor came out and asked me if I would come in when he talked with my wife. I asked him what was wrong and he said there was a cancerous tumor in her breast. My wife was sitting in the room when I entered and the doctor explained to both of us our options. I left the decision up to my wife as to whether to have a mastectomy or lumpectomy. I felt it was up to her to decide. Even at that time I did not think anything was going to happen to my wife. I felt it would be taken care of and everything would be fine. I did not realize the extensive procedures she was facing. I just thought this was going to be a routine procedure, and then everything was going to be fine.

My wife was scheduled for surgery and of course I went with her. I guess I still was in denial because I thought everything would be fine. She was being taken care of and God would take care of her. Nothing would happen to her.

HOPE

On Monday, May 17, she was going in to see her surgeon for results from the surgery. I went into work and then I thought to myself, "What am I doing here? I need to be with my wife." So I went to my supervisor and told him I was leaving because I needed to be with my wife for her appointment. I came home and my wife asked me what I was doing there. I said I am going with you. She told me I did not have to go but I said yes I do; I am going with you. I went into the operating room with my wife. Her doctor told her she did not have clear margins and that more surgery would be needed. I still did not believe anything would happen to my wife. I thought that she would be taken care of as more surgery was scheduled on Wednesday, May 19. Again I went with my wife. After surgery, the doctor came out and talked with me. I was told that he felt he had gotten everything this time and there was a clear margin. All the tissue would be sent to the lab for testing and he would let us know the results and another appointment would be scheduled. I went with my wife to her doctor appointment for results from the lab. We finally had clear margins. We were told radiation was the next step.

We were lucky enough to have a restful place to go. We had a camper set up on a permanent site where I would take her to rest and get away. The riding in the car was very difficult and painful for her from the surgeries. I tried to do my best to drive slowly, but it never seemed to be slow enough. Once we arrived at our campsite it was good and my wife was able to rest.

Radiation appointments were scheduled for my wife and I tried to get to every appointment with her. My wife took these appointments very well and never complained even though it was very frightening. I know the radiation caused her skin to be very uncomfortable. It was hard for her to put clothes on. It was hard for her to take a shower, but she never really complained about it. Thank goodness we had our camper to go to for relaxation and to get away from the stresses of it all. She was dealing with her boss, appointments and driving back and forth to work which was a long drive. But she did it and came through it very well.

About a year later she had to go for more surgery. She did not want me to go with her. She went alone. She was working, went into work, then left to go for the surgery. She did go back to work but her boss sent her home. My wife was very distraught. My wife felt ugly. I never looked at her that way. I felt she had not changed one bit. I did not understand how she could think that way. She had not changed one bit from the day I married her. I could not believe that she could look at herself that way. This last surgery changed my wife; she did not feel good about herself anymore.

What have helped both of us through this journey are the Oneida Area Cancer Support Group, Camp Good Days Women's Oncology program and Supportive Spouses weekends, and the American Cancer Society's I Can Cope series. At one I Can Cope meeting, a lady from Faxton-St. Lukes' Breast Care Center came and spoke about the services available to women who have had a mastectomy or lumpectomy. She met with my wife about the special undergarments available and since they met my wife has finally started to feel good about herself again.

We have met some wonderful people who are going through the very same thing and I am grateful to everyone for their support. I did not realize that this journey would be so difficult and so very hard. We have changed a lot of our ways, but we did it.

I would like to thank Patti McGee and Karen Litwak for being such good friends and having a support group that has saved a lot of people from a lot of unhappiness. I urge anyone who has any type of illness to find a support group, and I urge the caregiver to be with them. This journey should not be traveled alone. It is not just her illness; it is yours too. I feel we are some of the lucky ones. Thank you, God, most of all for helping us get through this.

Caregiver Poem
By Michael Counter

We honor the Caregivers
Who give so much of themselves.
For their loved ones.
When we were tired,
You were strong.
When they felt alone,
You did not leave.
When they gave in,
You did not give up.
When in pain they fell,
You loved them...
And their hearts could tell,
You were their Angel.

Family Caregiver
Karen McGee
Chadwicks, NY

I was first exposed to the word "cancer" when I was about 10-years-old. My girlfriend's 8-year-old little brother died of cancer and we all went to the calling hours but I didn't understand how awful it could be. About 28 years ago my girlfriend from Florida was diagnosed with breast cancer. Since she was miles away I still didn't grasp how horrible this can be for the patient until my best friend was diagnosed with cancer. I tried to help her by cooking, visiting and helping with holiday dinners for her and her family. It was very hard because she had lost her mother and two sisters to cancer within a few years of each other.

Then in 1994 my husband "Fibber" was diagnosed with prostate cancer. Prostate cancer, if caught early, has a high survival rate and the type of treatment was either surgery or radiation. My husband chose surgery and within a few weeks we were back golfing. I remember three weeks after the surgery he was still recuperating but wanted to go golfing. The doctor didn't want him to sit and ride in the golf cart so we came up with the plan that he would ride backwards in the golf cart and I would drive slowly. It was so funny to see him riding that way, but he was not going to let this hold him back. It has been 16 years that he has been cancer free. Although the initial diagnosis of my husband's cancer was very stressful, there was very little assistance needed as a caregiver. We celebrated our 50th wedding anniversary last year.

So in 2002, my daughter Patti was diagnosed with breast cancer and it really touched all of our family's lives. She began treatment in March of 2003 and I stayed with her and her 9-year-old son. He was so compassionate. The first night she was home from chemotherapy and was so ill with vomiting from the chemotherapy, he wiped her face down and emptied her puke bucket which he automatically did after each treatment.

When they are so ill you really don't think you are doing that much; but, it helps the patient just by being there. The best thing any caregiver can do is bring food, plants, cards, friendship and just your time but leave time for them to heal and grow on their own. To help anyone in need just be there to run errands, pick up medications and just show you care. One thing I learned while taking care of my daughter was not to hover over her. I had asked a neighbor to stay with her while I couldn't be there and my daughter called the neighbor and asked her not to come over that she would call her if she was needed because she felt I was hovering too much and needed space.

Side note from the Author:

Karen McGee is my mother and the support and love that she showed for my son Dylan and me was unconditional. The sacrifice she made to stay at my home to assist us during the week of my treatment to take care of me, cook and clean is so greatly appreciated. I believe that any illness will either bring a family closer together or put distance between them and it definitely brought the three of us closer. I will always cherish and be thankful for all she did and has done.

Dd - Determination

80 CB

Sometimes during diagnosis and treatment you may have to have a strong determination to help you get through. Take a picture of a loved one, your family or a pet, look at it daily and that will give you the determination that you need to get through.

As previously mentioned, a positive attitude plus determination will give you the strength to fight and feel that you can win this battle against cancer. If at any time during your treatment you feel distraught, tired or angry, reach out to your supporters and talk to them and let them help. I recommend seeking counseling just to give you someone you can talk to about how you are feeling if you do not feel like talking to a loved one or friend. Counseling has helped me tremendously throughout my journey. Sometimes talking to someone who doesn't know you as well as a friend or family member can help you see things in a better light or way.

A Family of Determination
By Flora Woodcock
Oneida, NY

In 2007 I was having some back pain but didn't think much about it because seven years prior I had had back surgery and thought maybe I did something to it again. I scheduled an appointment with my doctor and had some blood work and an MRI done. It was then in March of 2007 that I was diagnosed with acute myelogenous leukemia (AML). I was told to make an appointment with the hematologist to follow up with the blood work. The day I was scheduled with the hematologist, I received a phone call from them telling me that I would have to be admitted that day. I called my daughter and husband so they could drive me to the hospital and get me admitted to the oncology floor.

Everything was happening so fast. All the doctors started coming in and setting up IVs and they explained to my family that I was very sick and would be staying for quite some time. This is when I found out I had AML - a blood cancer. I personally don't remember being told because I was in so much pain. The doctors started chemotherapy right away. They had me on several different pain medications and nothing was touching the pain. I was unable to walk or get out of bed due to the pain I was in. This is when pneumonia set in. I started having problems breathing so I had to be put on a ventilator and was moved to the ICU unit where I spent the next ten weeks.

I was not able to receive any more chemotherapy treatments at this point due to being on the ICU unit. The doctors kept telling my family that I was a very sick woman and they were doing all they can. At one point they suggested to my family that maybe they should consider taking me off the ventilator and letting me go. The words the doctor said were, "You should stop doing things to her and doing things for her." My family decided to have a family meeting with the doctors to discuss all the options.

The first question asked by the family was what is the status of the AML? The oncologist stated that it was in remission.

Although we knew the family was going to continue fighting, they also continued to gather more information. I was on the vent unit for approximately eight weeks. My family prayed, read get well cards and letters that were sent and of course had faith. Shortly after the decision was made to keep fighting, I started getting better and they were able to start weaning me off the ventilator.

Once I was off the vent and continued with more chemotherapy treatments, the doctors stated that I was going to need a bone marrow transplant to survive. My two sisters were tested, but were not matches and my daughters were not eligible to be matches so they wouldn't test them. I was then referred to Roswell Park Cancer Institute. I went to Buffalo, NY to meet with Dr. McCarthy, a bone marrow specialist. He gave us all the information about the benefits and risks and explained the procedure. Although it is not an easy procedure, my will to live was much stronger so I decided to seek out a donor. Finding a donor can take anywhere from six weeks to six months and sometimes a donor is never found. I received a call in seven weeks to say they found a perfect match, ten out of ten. Thank you Lord; our prayers were answered. I was told to be in Buffalo on December 5 to start the process. I had to go through another round of chemotherapy and then on December 12, I had the transplant. It was amazing that a little bag of stem cells from a complete stranger could save your life. I thank God for the wonderful people who are willing to be donors. You are unable to have contact for the first year with the donor so I was only told that it was a 30-year old male. At the end of one year, I was able to contact and thank the young man who helped save my life.

During my sickness I had a good attitude. Yes, I had bad days; that is normal. But I do believe if you have strong faith and also have a positive attitude it helps you. My husband, daughters, family, friends, pastor and our church family, along with the doctors and nurses were all wonderful and very helpful throughout my journey. The unsettling thing about cancer is that it can strike anyone at any time, no matter how much you exercise, or how good a person you are. It's like a bolt out of the blue. Fortunately the medical profession is making progress.

This has been a difficult journey, but the people who have been there for me have been overwhelming.   Thank you for all your prayers and support. Keep a POSITIVE ATTITUDE and remember Matthew 19-Verse 26, "With God all things are possible." We have started a team for the Leukemia Society's "MIRACLE IN MOTION" fundraiser because that is what I truly am.

"All the Wonders that you seek are within yourself" - Sir Thomas Browne

Ee - Exercise

ℰℭ

Daily exercise is very important. It helps to keep a positive attitude and will also help you feel better. Your physical ability will determine the type of exercise and the duration. Make sure you check with your doctor before beginning any exercise routine.

Exercise will help keep your mind off your treatment and will help with fatigue that sometimes can really frustrate you. Some sample exercises that other survivors have mentioned that helped them are: breathing, arm stretches, leg lifts, yoga and tai chi.

Buddy up to exercise with another survivor. You will be more dedicated if you have someone to exercise with and you won't find yourself making excuses for why you can't exercise.

Massage therapy is also a good outlet for healing your mind and body. I had scar tissue from my partial mastectomy and was introduced to a massage therapist and she helped me through some of my most stressful times of my life. One special type of massage that I like to use on my clients is called facilitated stretching. Facilitated stretching allows the therapist to determine if the client has tight fascia (skin) or scar tissue that is inhibiting the person to stretch. Through the use of massage you can lengthen short and contracted muscles and contract overstretched and weak muscles.

I do recommend that if you do receive massage therapy you seek out a therapist who has experience in working with people dealing with cancer.

Ride of Your Life
Exercise, Faith and Love
Bill Wiley
Sherrill, NY

I was diagnosed on May 20, 2005 with Stage IV colon cancer having gone to my liver and at first I was devastated, shocked and scared. I thought I was going to die within 2 to 3 years. With the help of a lot of people in the medical field both at the Oneida Oncology Group and Memorial Sloan Kettering and with the help of prayers to a very forgiving God from people I don't even know, I am still here to tell my story.

I was in good shape at the time of my diagnosis and I continued to try to work out. I turned my running and swimming into swimming, biking and running. My son and I trained for the NYC Triathlon and completed it three times; the last time my daughter joined us.

Cancer has changed my life completely. As an avid runner to stay in shape after my diagnosis, I began running back to the one aspect of my life I had been running from and I accepted Jesus Christ as my Savior. I put Him in complete control of my life.

My family was totally awesome. My wife Donna was the best caregiver anyone could ask for. My daughter was always there with medical help; she is an M.D. My son was my research specialist on the Internet and actually was the first person to suggest I go to Dr. Nancy Kemeny for treatment in NYC. My youngest daughter prayed and told me God had told her I was going to be a miracle.

My friends have rallied behind me. My friends in Sherrill continue to push me to run, swim and bike with them. My childhood friends that I grew up with now live all over the country. They bought bikes and camping gear and trained to ride a yearly bike tour with me. We have done three tours that consist of biking as much as 95 miles in a day and setting up camp in tents. Then we pack up the next day and ride someplace else. Our tours are up to 6 days long and we average 60 to 65 miles a day. These are guys I played Pop Warner football with and we still are great friends who love to hang together. Oh, by the way, we start each morning ride in prayer.

Dr. Kemeny told me that exercise keeps the tumors away. She was always supportive of me continuing to live a very active life. Exercise has always been a part of my life but I gained strength from my cancer diagnosis. I recommend that you get into shape so you can be your best in battle. You are now on the championship field. Your opponent is TOUGH. You have two options: fold, give up, and lose OR fight the best fight that you can. Make Jesus your coach; make the doctors your quarterback. Get in the trenches and battle. Have a game plan and follow it. That is all you can do.

Remember that no one knows what is around the corner. Don't wait too long to realize that your only way to Heaven is through Jesus Christ who died to save you from sins that you can never repay. Also you will find your strength in your family and your REAL friends; beware of the ones who say they are but aren't. Over the years, I realized that God was in complete control of my life and death. He has a plan for me and my closest friends and relatives. I am not afraid of death because I know what awaits me after my time here on earth. I know that when it comes it will be because my work has been completed here and I am being called home to be with my Savior.

Since my diagnosis I am now loving life; I am about to become a grandfather with both my girls pregnant at the same time. I am about to become a father-in-law for the third time. My son is marrying a wonderful girl whom we love.

I would encourage you to read the Bible and Lance Armstrong's book "It's Not About the Bike" to help you through your journey.

A special thanks to my wife Donna who has stuck with me through good times and bad. She is a rock of strength. She has always loved me unconditionally even when I had her driving all over Oneida looking for root beer popsicles. The nursing staff at the oncology group always tried to keep me laughing during my treatments. I would also like to thank the doctors and staff at the Oneida Oncology Group and at Memorial Sloan Kettering. I am alive today to enjoy my family, faith and love due to them, for that I will be eternally grateful. I am a very lucky man.

Ff - Family
෯ఴ

Reach out to family and friends. You will be touched by many new friends who have gone through or are going through the same experiences. Embrace them. You will also strengthen and renew family ties with members of your immediate family. There is no greater bond than that of a strong family and friendship.

As you go through your journey with cancer, remember that your family is also going through it themselves. It is important to talk to them and let them know what they can do to help you. I remember when I was going through my treatment, my father and my brother Shawn did not know how to help me or talk to me. I remember telling my brother Shawn, the two men in my life, ran the other way and he looked at me and said, "You are right." From that day forward he was himself and I knew that if I ever needed anything I could call him.

Remember family and real friends accept us as we are and see the best in us.

One Loving Family
Linda G.
Rome, NY

It was Thanksgiving time when my family and I were celebrating everything in life that we were thankful for: two wonderful children, two grandchildren and my husband and

I being married for 33 years. I have always made sure that my family and I had our yearly physicals and exams. It is part of the perfectionist in me and so I had recently made my yearly mammogram for that November. At my routine appointment, the technician noticed an abnormality, and after consulting with my doctor a biopsy was scheduled with lymph node removal. Although it was a very trying time between the mammogram and the surgery, I tried to remain optimistic and my family was extremely supportive. The day of surgery I made my doctor, whom I love dearly, promise to tell me the results if she knew after the surgery because I trusted her and wanted to hear from her. It was at that time I was diagnosed with triple negative metastatic ductal carcinoma breast cancer.

With my family by my side, I remember how scared, shocked and numb I became as my doctor was telling us about my diagnosis. My biggest fear was for my family, especially my husband and my son who has Down syndrome. I also started wondering if I would get to see my grandchildren grow up. There are so many fears and worries that go through your mind.

As I went through treatment, I remember how in the "Chemo Lounge" there was no computer for patient use and the television was very old. As a family, we have all learned how life can change at any moment. In keeping with our family philosophy to give back to our community, we decided to donate a computer for the chemotherapy lounge at the oncology center. We raised money at family gatherings by holding raffles and donating loose change. After one year my family raised enough money to purchase a computer. I was also fortunate to win a local television contest that was part of Oprah Winfrey's "Big Give" and I was able to donate a big screen television. I submitted an essay about how the TV at the oncology center was old and it would be nice to have something to watch while going through treatment. Being able to give back helped me to deal with my cancer and was part of the healing process after treatment.

Through the treatment process my family, especially my husband, was always there for me. We have learned to celebrate life's little moments as well as the big ones. I kept a journal and in it I wrote down everything I was thankful for: the times my husband rubbed my bald head so I could get some sleep; talking to my daughter every day; the times my son tucked me into bed and kissed my cheek; and for being able to read to my grandchildren because we never know what tomorrow is going to bring.

As time has gone by, instead of being a cancer victim I now celebrate each year that I am a survivor. My grandchildren gave me a pink heart earring and I wear it faithfully in the upper part of my ear. The second year I got a butterfly tattoo, something I would have never done prior to being diagnosed with cancer. I chose a butterfly because it represents how short life can be and it is a reminder to live life to its fullest.

If I could reach out to another cancer patient, I would encourage them to journal and keep notes of doctor's appointments, symptoms they are having and what they are thankful for in life. Make sure you eat ice cream to celebrate the small victories such as after each chemotherapy treatment and each day of survivorship.

Although I had an aggressive cancer and have been able to beat it, I never could have done it without the love and support of the people closest to me: MY FAMILY.

Stay positive; you can beat it too!!

Gg - Gutsy
∞∞

Many family members and friends will tell you how courageous you are as you go through your treatments. There may be times during your treatment that you will feel like you have had enough and do not want to continue; talk to your doctor and see if he or she can postpone a treatment and give you an extra week in between. Once around the 5th or 6th treatment we had to postpone it to give my body time to recuperate. I was experiencing dehydration, I had double eye infections, and a chest infection as my chemotherapy built up and my immune system weakened. It is very common, so don't get frustrated.

One of my most favorite places to attend is Camp Good Days and Special Times in Upstate NY. It started out as a camp for children with cancer and has expanded to include adult oncology programs but on the back of the tee shirts they hand out to campers it reads "Where Courage knows no boundaries." You will find the strength to beat this disease.

Staying Positive
Donna Wallace
Canastota, NY

I am a 17 year breast cancer survivor. Eleven years before I was diagnosed with breast cancer, my sister Ann died at the age of 42 from breast cancer. From that point on, at the age of 36, I went every year for a mammogram. At the age of 47, I felt a lump in my left breast while showering.

Six months before I found my lump I was having problems with my period; I was bleeding all the time. I went to a local doctor and he put me on a hormone pill. I had expressed concern and told him about my sister Ann dying of breast cancer but he said this pill was okay. Well six months later I had breast cancer. My cancer doctor told me it did not cause my cancer but activated it. So if you have a family history of breast cancer please research the idea about taking a hormone pill. It's harder to go through menopause with hot flashes and other side effects but it's not that bad considering the risk of hormone replacement for people with a family history of cancer.

After I found my lump, I went for a mammogram and sonogram and then was referred to Dr. Kelly. He said all it showed were cysts. I had cysts in both breasts. He tried to aspirate one of the cysts and decided I would need a biopsy because there was no fluid from the aspiration. We scheduled a hysterectomy and the biopsy for the same time. The biopsy showed cancer in both breasts. Dr. Kelly saved my life. Three weeks after my biopsy I had a double mastectomy and had all my lymph nodes removed on both sides.

Throughout all of this my very special husband and best friend Gerald was there for me every step of the way. When we got home from the hospital he said, "What do you want to do? I said I want to sit on the couch and have you look at this. He did and he said "What's the problem; you're alive aren't you?" I chose not to have reconstructive surgery and his attitude is still the same today.

I had six months of chemotherapy, two weeks on two weeks off for a total of 12 treatments. On the weeks I had chemotherapy I felt crappy for a couple days and just slept. I worked through the last four months of treatment.

I had some good days and bad days. My best friend Jean had a mastectomy four months before me and she was my rock! She would call me every day and ask me if it was going to be a bad day or a good day. Most days I would say a good day. We both love the sunshine; it made us feel better so now we go to Florida for the winter.

The way I got through my first year was to talk about my cancer. When Jean and I were going through it there was no support group available. Now we have a wonderful support group. You leave there feeling good.

When I would get blue, my husband and I would go visit our neighbors who had their 2-year-old granddaughter living with them and she would make me laugh. So please get out of the house and see someone that will make you laugh. Also get out in the sunshine; it will make you feel better. Just remember there is a light at the end of the tunnel. Please try to keep a positive attitude. I think that is how you heal.

Please try not to sweat the little stuff. Things that might have bothered me before cancer don't anymore. I try to help people who are going through a rough time. Please take time to smell the roses. Take time for family and friends; you won't regret it. It will make you feel wonderful.

I dedicate this story to my husband Gerald, my sons, Scott and Dick, and my best friend, Jean.

"Strength does not come from physical capacity;
It comes from an indomitable will." - Mahatma Gandhi

Hh - Hug
ଽ෮ଽ

In today's society we do not take the time to hug and embrace those important and special to us. You will meet many special people; embrace them with open arms.

You will be going through a healing process not only from surgery or side effects from treatment but mentally from the diagnosis. Let those closest to you know you appreciate their support by just giving them a gentle hug.

I believe a hug a day will help keep the doctor and the blues away.

Knowing Your Body
Michele Doeing
Liverpool, NY

In the winter of 2007 I noticed that the mole on the back of my leg was rubbing on my clothing and bothered me so I went to my doctor. My doctor looked it over and said it was nothing but if I wanted it removed we could do it. I decided to leave it alone and thought nothing of it for about eight months then I decided it should be removed because it was still bothering me. My doctor scheduled the surgery for the day before Thanksgiving and after removing it she said she removed it all and would contact me if there were any problems.

On December 11, 2007 I received a phone call from my doctor telling me that my mole was cancerous, called dermatofibrosarcoma protuberans (DFSP) and she did not get a clear margin and I would have to have more surgery. I remember my doctor asking me if I was okay and made sure I understood what she had said. I next remember talking on the phone to my husband as he was coming home from work. I tried to pretend that nothing was wrong but he could sense there was and convinced me to tell him; I really didn't want to tell him over the phone. I remember telling him I would talk to him when he came home because I really just wanted to be alone to take it all in and learn to cope. As I cried, I remember thinking I am the strong one; I need to take care of everyone else just like in 2006 when my husband had his heart attack. When my husband came home he just hugged me and we cried. I remember him wanting to be close to me, but I really wanted to be alone to try and digest that I had cancer.

My doctor had recommended that I see a dermatologist the next day and when I arrived the nurse did not even know why I was there and had never heard of DFSP. I really didn't feel comfortable with their office and sought out another surgeon in Rochester, NY. Doctor G. told me I was going to need Mohs surgery which would remove the tumor and give them a clear margin; they removed a tumor the size of a plum along with two other moles. I have scar tissue in my leg but with Mohs surgery, they spare the healthy tissue and only remove the cancerous tissue so I am confident they removed it all. Due to the high recurrence rate, I have to have full body scans every six months and have been taught the proper way to scan my body for any changes in my moles.

HOPE

Through all of this, the support I have received from my
family, friends and coworkers has been unbelievable. My
daughter was there every day taking care of me and my
boss and coworkers were very supportive. When I
returned to work all my coworkers hugged me and
welcomed me back, they raised money to help pay for tolls,
gas and surgery. I was so thankful for all the support I
received.

ii - Inspiration
ଧୋଓଃ

You are going to meet some special individuals who are going to inspire you to keep going and you will also inspire others to keep going through discussing your experiences with them. Don't be afraid to open up and share your fears and experiences; it will be beneficial to others and yourself.

I have found that by attending local support groups you can be an inspiration to other survivors whether it is with a hug, sharing your journey and experiences or just by sitting and listening to them. I suggest you contact your local oncology office or the American Cancer Society for information on support groups in your area.

Seven years ago, my oncology nurse practitioner and I started a monthly support group and an I Can Cope series in conjunction with the American Cancer Society and we still facilitate it today. The I Can Cope series is a four week educational series where we bring in doctors and other speakers to talk about topics to help individuals move on in an area that they may be struggling with since their treatment. At one series, we brought in a speaker from the Faxton-St. Luke's Breast Care Center's Perfect Fit Boutique in Utica, NY to talk about the services that are offered. After telling us about how to get fitted for a new bra after a partial or full mastectomy, I remember one of the survivors coming up to me after the meeting and telling me with tears in her eyes that she thought there was no hope for her to feel whole again and that she had an appointment the next day. The next day I was at work, and later that afternoon, in comes the survivor with the biggest smile on her face and with tears streaming down her face she shows me her new bra and gives me the biggest hug and thanks me for bringing the speaker out. It is moments like that inspire me to keep offering the programs.

Faith, Strength and Support
Leo Matzke
Oneida, NY

My journey with cancer began in May of 1989. I went to the doctors to check out a small amount of bleeding coming from the rectum. I went thinking I had hemorrhoids, but came away knowing I had a very large cancerous tumor. I still remember the doctor pulling my wife aside and telling her we're in big trouble. That, maybe, I had two months to live.

I was immediately sent to a surgeon at University Hospital. After a consultation, it was decided that the tumor was too big and needed to be shrunk before surgery could take place. So during the summer of 1989, I went for radiation treatments which did in fact shrink and kill the tumor. Surgery took place in September of that year but during surgery, the surgeon saw that I had cancer elsewhere, particularly throughout my liver. Because the tumor was so close to the end of my rectum, that part of my body had to be removed so I was left with a permanent colostomy. Things looked very bleak once again.

It was at that time that my wife and I were approached to see if we were willing to be part of an experimental group for advanced colon cancer patients. Up until that time, advanced colon cancer was almost always fatal. We jumped at the chance. After 10 months of chemotherapy with experimental drugs, the surgeon felt that the tumors in my liver had shrunk and could be removed. She went back in, removed about a third of my liver, scraped several other of my internal organs, and I'm still here today.

Five years later, colon cancer appeared in my right lung. Again, it didn't look good but after some convincing, the radiologists were willing to use radiology to kill the tumors in my right lung. After another six months of chemotherapy, they performed the radiology treatment, and although the treatment burned the lower two lobes of my right lung, the therapy did kill the tumors. Although I can't say I'm cancer free, I can say I'm in full remission and have been so for 15 years now.

I would like to conclude by pointing out five things:

First, this disease is as hard on the caregiver as it is on the caretaker. This was very hard on my wife and three children. My wife is my rock and I've never seen her so scared. It also took a terrible toll on my children. They felt lost. All a caregiver can do is worry, and that makes them feel so helpless at a time when they want to be very supportive.

Second, my faith was a strong part in helping me get through the ordeal. I would pretend that I had my head in Jesus' lap and He would reach into my body and pluck out the cancer cells. Believe it or not, I got this image from watching a mother monkey plucking lice off her babies. Funny how that came about. But knowing Christ was there for me brought great comfort.

Third, when this happened, I was a teacher. My students and fellow staff members gave me great support. The students somehow understood, for they became angels and we're talking 6th graders; they're never angels. I would teach Monday through Thursday and go into the hospital every Friday for my eight-hour chemo drip.

Fourth, seeing my name on several prayer lists gave me great strength. Knowing that there were people out there who were supporting me even though they didn't know me and that we were all in this together gave me a sense of great hope.

Lastly, I knew the doctors and nurses were pulling for me. Their mannerism made me feel that we were all part of one team and my success was their goal.

"The Sun shines not on us, but in us" - John Muir

Jj - Journaling
80 03

In looking back through the book as I have written it, I realize that journaling was such a big part of my healing process and journey. Each letter represents how I was feeling or how I was able to help someone else through their journey. As I read through my journal and see how I have evolved from being scared, frustrated and feeling guilty because I have survived while others have passed away, to taking what I have learned and passing it on to other cancer survivors through support groups, massage therapy and most of all the gift of listening, I see how beneficial journaling truly is.

Journaling will help you in many ways. Keeping track of how you feel will help let your doctor know what is bothering you. By writing it down you won't have to try and remember everything you need to discuss with your doctor.

Journaling can also help you write down your feelings and help to get any anger or frustration out. Your journaling can be kept secret where only you know what you have written or you can share your experiences with your loved ones and friends. It is a great way to get rid of any anxiety and frustration. Usually once you have written in your journal and then you reflect back on it as time passes, you think "Why was I so stressed or angry over that? It really wasn't that big of a deal."

My main focus in writing the book is to help someone who might be struggling with their diagnosis or side effects of the medications know that they are not alone; there is someone else out there that has gone through it or is going through it. When I was first diagnosed, I didn't have a clue where to begin. I trusted my doctors and with the help of family and friends, I got through it. Most of my journey began after my chemotherapy and radiation treatments ended and it was time to move on. I was thrust into menopause and my body was fighting it along with my mind. There were days I didn't know if I could keep going. I would just look at my son and say just one more day, just give yourself one more day. Now it has been seven years and I am writing a book. What a journey. I still journal when I need to but as time passes, I find it gets less and less each year.

Through our support groups and I Can Cope series we offer journaling as part of the programs. We have guest speakers give presentations on journaling and hand out journals to get started. The American Cancer Society also has booklets and journals so do not hesitate to contact them to get started.

Journaling, meditation and proper breathing techniques help to calm the body, mind and spirit and bring your body back to feeling whole. I encourage you to keep journaling as long as it takes to help you through your journey with cancer.

"Happiness is found along the way not at the end of the road." Author Unknown

By Joyce E. Walker
Verona, NY

Sterile walls start staring back
Urging me to think attack.
Radiation, chemo, pills
Vibrate nerves and give me chills.
Inside, outside I can see
Visions rise in front of me.
On a wing my angels fly --
Rise to heaven, live or die.

A SURVIVOR I must be --
DAYS or YEARS -- I'm CANCER-FREE!!!

Kk - Knowledge
ಕೂಡ

Knowledge is power so learn as much as you can about your disease or illness and educate yourself on the types of treatment available to you. The more knowledge you have about your treatment the stronger you will be throughout it.

A good place to start is the American Cancer Society. The American Cancer Society has information on all types of cancers and also has many support programs to help you through your journey. You can access the American Cancer Society online at www.cancer.org or at 1-800-227-2345.

Your local oncology department should give you information on the treatment and drugs you will be given along with any side effects of the medications.

If you have any doubts and want further information, get a second opinion or seek out survivors who can talk to you about what helped them through their treatment.

"Learning is a lifelong experience"
Julie Hanna (2007 Lessons for Life Calendar)

Life's Lessons
Aimee Gasparre
Rochester, NY

On December 23, 2003, my world was rocked. At a routine mammogram, I pointed out an area to the radiologist that I wasn't very concerned about because it wasn't hard, round, or pea-like as I always was taught to look for. As I spent more and more hours getting an ultrasound and then a core biopsy, my fear rose. My doctor told me she was very concerned about what she was seeing. I was shocked and scared. I was all by myself, which was ironic since I was always so nervous during my mammograms that my best friend and I had decided to start going together the following year. This would have been my last one alone. When I got the news that it was indeed cancer I felt immobilized. My knees actually shook. It was truly surreal.

I gave myself two days to fall apart. Then I decided I had to take some action so I could get some control of it all. I read all I could so I was able to make more informed choices. I called a friend who had been through it and asked a lot of questions. I started to realize that cancer didn't equal a death sentence. I went to the bookstore with my sisters and bought several books including **Just Get Me Through This!: The Practical Guide to Breast Cancer** by Deborah A. Cohen.

For several months I felt like I was constantly buzzing, like no place felt comfortable or safe. The biggest thing I found myself doing was trying to take ownership of everyone's feelings. When I had to tell a friend or co-worker that I had cancer, I would just say "I have breast cancer. But I am fine!" I tried to take their fear away immediately. It became exhausting to do that and I finally recognized that it was okay for people who cared about me to be concerned and a little frightened. I started setting boundaries, though. I did not want to hear about everyone's aunt, cousin, sister, friend or mother who had breast cancer and their treatments and their outcomes. But if they insisted, it had to have a happy ending. Most people understood that. Some didn't.

I am an artistic and musical person by nature. But I felt like I was living in white. I had no colors in me. That lasted for about eight months. Slowly, I started re-emerging. That's when I started feeling my sense of self return. That, and when my hair started growing back. I stopped wearing scarves when it was about 1/8" long. At first, I wore wigs that were not like my own short dark hair at all. It was actually fun for a little while. But then, I had enough of feeling like I was an imposter.

One of the biggest changes I made was to take strict control of my diet. I read **Beating Cancer with Nutrition** by Patrick Quillen. I started following **The pH Miracle Diet: Balance Your Diet, Reclaim Your Health** by Robert O. **Young** and Shelley Redford **Young,** which emphasizes eating alkaline-based foods rather than acid based. I gave up sugar, white flour and dairy products. I concentrated on greens, veggies, citrus fruits, fiber rich carbohydrates, almond butter and almond cheese. I actually never felt better in my life. I strongly feel that sugar feeds cancer cells and did all I could to eliminate it from my diet.

My life lessons have been great. I have become a sort of go-to person for women who have either been diagnosed or have a loved one or friend who's been diagnosed. I've been able to help people get started on this uninvited journey, and to breathe a little. I sometimes wonder if I was diagnosed so I can help guide others through it when they need some help. I have met remarkable women who have lived with such adversity, including repeated bouts of ovarian or breast cancer that has spread, but they keep moving forward, keep on living their lives even with these fierce "interruptions". I truly try to live the Serenity Prayer; changing what I can, accepting the things I can't, and having the wisdom to know the difference. It is not always easy. But I think it's essential to my well being.

There definitely were some funny and outrageous moments through this journey. One of the key ones was when I was driving home from work in 80+ degree weather with my air conditioner not working and just miserable with my itchy wig. When I couldn't stand it one more minute, I tore it off and threw it into the back seat. I then happened to glance at a guy in the car next to me staring at me with his eyes huge, and about to drive off the road.

I use April 23 as my "cancerversary" date, being the day I had surgery, not the day I was diagnosed. I am now a six year cancer survivor. Reaching five years was a very powerful milestone for me. I now try to give back to those who gave to me by volunteering for places such as Camp Good Days & Special Times, which is a camp for children with cancer, but also has adult oncology weekends. My husband and I help out quite a bit for their Finger Lakes International Wine Competition and auction. I advocate for others when possible. Not just for cancer survivors but for those who are being wronged. I try to choose words more carefully, and think how they could affect others. I try to live in a way that gives my life purpose. I know unbelievable and wonderful women because of my diagnosis and I am so grateful to have them in my life. I am touched by people such as my pottery class teacher, a breast cancer survivor who holds a free class for other survivors, just charging for supplies. She is a remarkable and kind person and because of her, more women have become part of my breast cancer network. I will never stop being overwhelmed by the amount of people I know who have been directly or indirectly touched by cancer. I feel like I am more hopeful that cancer will be able to be prevented in the future, than that there will be an actual cure. With the countless numbers of different cancers and scenarios for each diagnosis, I'm not sure how realistic a cure would be.

For someone newly diagnosed, my advice is to allow yourself a day or two to freak out, and then start taking all the action you can. Line up your doctors; build your support team. Become informed. Ask questions. Take each step one at a time. Read what you need to know, then put the book away and digest the information. Don't spend too much time researching on the Internet. It can be a very scary place. Go to sites such as www.breastcancer.org for online support groups. They have groups for newly diagnosed people, those having chemo, those having radiation, and those who are past treatment.

It's imperative to have a positive feel for your team of doctors. Make sure you interview a couple of surgeons, because one will probably fit you better than another. It was important to me that they were not only informative and direct, but that they treated me as an individual, not just another person with cancer. I had a strong and knowledgeable team who was able to be compassionate and listen to me when I had questions or was afraid or needed to cry. I wanted someone who respected that I intended to incorporate some holistic treatment such as acupuncture and massage therapy along with Western medicine. At first, there are so many questions that run through your mind when you go to your various doctors. Have one notebook to write them down in so that you'll remember to ask them. I suggest you take someone close to you to all appointments, who is also a pretty good note taker (and uses your notebook). Your head will probably be swirling with all the information you will be receiving.

Many of us refer to this as a journey. It will have some positive sides that will surprise you, if you keep your heart and mind open. Sometimes it takes a long time for you to realize this. But you will move forward when you are ready. You will meet some amazing people who touch you and change you. You will find kindness in unlikely places. And you will give back if you're able. With love and light, I wish healing and peace to you all.

LL - Live, Laugh and Love
∞∞

These three words will inspire you to stay strong, cherish every moment and embrace those important to you.

If you haven't already started, take a good look at your life and start living it to the fullest. The old proverb said "laughter is the best medicine." Surround yourself with only loving individuals, they help to keep you strong.

As the co-chair of two cancer support groups I've heard many of the participants talk about how they are not the same people they were before their diagnosis. They appreciate life more and worry less about the small things in life that happen.

Laughter is known to help cheer you up and get your blood flowing, so rent a good movie and enjoy it.

"Life is a dance when you take the steps"
Author Unknown

Cancer "Sucks"
By Lisa Thomas
Hamilton, NY

It was late in August 2003 when my husband, three sons and I were getting ready to go to North Carolina and Georgia to look for employment. My husband was looking for a new job so we decided the best thing for our family would be to move down south. We had the car packed and left our sons with my parents while my husband and I went to get the results of my tests, figuring I would just run in and get a clean bill of health and then be on our way to start over.

I remember the doctor coming into the room and looking at me and saying those small but powerful words, "It's malignant which means cancer." I immediately went into shock and disbelief. I also feared for my children, wondering if I was going to be alive for their next birthday, and what they would do without me. I thought, "I am only 33-years-old."

Over the next couple years there was much uncertainty. I became very depressed. I wondered if I could have any more children and struggled going from day to day. I isolated myself from my loved ones but they stayed strong and were my rock. My sister Laura and my family were with me from start to finish. She sought other cancer survivors for me to talk to and was very patient with me.

It is hard for children to understand the changes you are going through due to the side effects of chemotherapy, losing your hair and being tired all the time. I remember my son Spencer who was 18 months old at the time had a hard time seeing me with no hair and when I would get a hot flash and take off my cap he would say "Hat on Mommy, Hat on!" It would always make me laugh.

In September 2005, I wasn't feeling well and I went to the doctor and found out I was pregnant with our 4th child and another boy. Again, I began to fear if he would be okay after I had the chemotherapy and had just recently stopped taking tamoxifin. I had a test done in December and it showed a healthy boy. I was relieved. Kayden is now 4-years-old and still a typical healthy boy.

Over the years I have learned who my true friends are and I feel I have become a stronger person. The friends I thought I could count on to help me through my journey somehow vanished and those I never expected to be there were always there and became my support and my best friends. I try not to take things for granted but cherish what I do have: friends, family and love. I definitely have become more aware of my surroundings.

Through all the pain and anguish I have learned that life isn't always what it seems and can change in an instant. My life has changed and I will never be the same as before I was diagnosed. I view things differently, and feel different both mentally and physically. There will always be uncertainty in my life wondering if all the aches and pains are the cancer returning but over the years it has become less and less.

If I could help someone else who was recently diagnosed with cancer, I would tell them to research their cancer; find out everything about all their options for treatment and to attend a support group. I have met so many wonderful people through our local cancer support group, the American Cancer Society's Relay For Life and Camp Good Days and Special Times.

"Cancer Sucks!!!" But the friends that I made through this emotional and physical journey make you wonder the reason things happen.

Mon - Medication
ℰᎧᏟᏰ

The medications and drugs that the doctors use during your treatment can have side effects. It is very important for you to let your doctor know how you are feeling if something doesn't seem right. During your treatment and after, you may have to go on an antidepressant to help rebalance your mind and body. This is okay; do not feel like you are weak or helpless. It takes time to heal and part of the healing process is how to manage your life mentally. Talk to your doctor and develop a plan for treatment.

After I finished my chemotherapy and radiation, my doctor recommended I take tamoxifin for five years to help prevent the cancer from recurring. I started the tamoxifin in September and by November that year I remember calling the oncology office crying. I was telling the nurse practitioner that I couldn't stop crying and I was sitting in front of my refrigerator eating a box of Hostess Ho-Ho's. She asked me if I was suicidal. I told her no, but that I couldn't stop crying and I didn't know what was going on. She told me to stop taking the tamoxifin, because I was having side effects from it. I went off it for a few months and we tried it again but I started having the same side effects so we stopped it all together. My next choice was to be put into menopause and use arimadex along with lupron. The combination of the two medications caused the same type of side effects and I had to stop that treatment. My doctor told me because I was not at a menopausal age my body did not like the hormones. We let my body get rid of the medications and heal and then we tried a third hormonal treatment called femara but about six months into the treatment, I started having the same symptoms and stopped taking the medication. I am called "My problem child" by my oncologist.

If you have concerns or questions about the medications you are taking there are two websites that can assist you www.consumermedsafety.org and www.safemedication.com. These two websites can report medication errors, guide you on how to administer your medication, and are there to protect you from drug interactions.

"Memories help us celebrate the past,
Live in the present
And hold hope for the future.
Share memories with those you love"
Julie Hanna

Keep it Light!
By Mike Healy
Oneida, NY

It was in 1980 as I lay in my hospital bed on a blustery March day in Central New York. I had completed my "beloved" sponge bath, had breakfast and was now anxiously awaiting the true highlight of my day, the arrival of my favorite visitor, my wife Colleen. I couldn't wait to share my "big revelation" with my best friend!

First, let's back up a bit. In October we had celebrated the arrival of our first child, Gillian Beth. Then, one month to the day later, Colleen's father died of a heart attack while deer hunting. Talk about an emotional roller coaster! And if that wasn't enough, in the days that followed, I noticed some numbness in my left leg and thought I better let my doctor know. The next morning, I'm in the office of a neurologist and one test after another is being ordered. I was admitted to the hospital later that day and wouldn't come home for two weeks. Poor Colleen never even had a chance to mourn her father's death, what with a month-old baby and now this! I was diagnosed with a malignant fibrous histiocytoma (MFH), also called giant cell sarcoma of the soft tissue.

In a planned approach, the first part of the tumor that had been discovered would be removed from within my spinal column by a neurosurgeon and, three months later, the other part would be removed from the back wall of my chest cavity by a thoracic surgeon. I was now recovering from that surgery and was experiencing all the pain that goes with such a procedure, especially when the respiratory therapists would put me through my deep breathing exercises. And then there was the coughing; every one a new "adventure" that I truly dreaded although I understood the importance of keeping my lungs clear.

Little did we know at the time, but those procedures signaled the beginning of a nearly twenty-year saga that would include eight more major operations - some less than two years apart - to either remove recurrences of the tumor or reconstruct areas that had been compromised by skin grafting and radiation therapy. The biggest procedure of all involved removal of about forty percent of the soft tissue in my back, removal of several vertebrae and fusing of the spine, all of which left me somewhat compromised structurally, not to mention a few inches shorter.

I've been blessed with a terrific wife who has been with me through all of the procedures, all the worrying, all the waiting and all the wondering. She has changed her share of dressings over the years and has had to deal with far more than I would ever wish on anyone. She was with me when the surgeon uttered those dreaded words: "It's malignant." She was with me when another doctor advised: "Get your affairs in order and plan for the children's education because you probably won't be around for that." (Our other daughter, Claire, was born about two and a half years after Gillian.) The girls have also seen and experienced more than children should ever have to.

Through it all and for reasons I can't fully explain, I have always been able to keep a positive, upbeat attitude and even find humor in the cards life has dealt me (us). The way I look at it, there's always someone else who's worse off than I am. Spending many days and nights in intensive care drives that home in a hurry. Quite honestly, the biggest problem I've had is being less than completely sensitive to the fact that Colleen, and most normal people for that matter, doesn't necessarily share my fatalistic and somewhat cavalier approach to some pretty serious matters. And I would get very uncomfortable and even annoyed by being around people who took my situation much more seriously that I cared to. I'm a firm believer that life is twenty percent what happens to you and eighty percent how you deal with what happens to you. Like I said, I don't know why I'm like that and it certainly isn't that I'm in denial. I'm just convinced that everyone has to find their own way of dealing with adversity. What works for me doesn't necessarily work for others and I have really had to work on trying to be more sensitive and respectful of other people's ways of handling difficult situations and expressing their concern.

Frankly, it's hard to get too down on things when I've managed to stay around to see Gillian and Claire graduate from college and become an elementary teacher and surgical RN, respectively. More recently, Gillian married a great guy and made us extremely proud grandparents of a handsome baby boy who is the light of "Nana's & Papa's" lives. (Remember, I wasn't expected to be around for all of these milestones!) I'm able to maintain a productive career, go fishing with good friends and enjoy a fairly normal life, so who am I to complain? Indeed, this book is filled with the stories of many people who have endured much more than I have and are far more courageous than I'll ever be. I wish them well because we're all "Kindred Spirits" of sorts.

So, what was that "big revelation" that I mentioned way back in the opening paragraph? Well, during those dreaded respiratory therapy sessions, it was painfully obvious (literally) just how limited and weak my coughs were, which struck me as very funny. So much so that I couldn't wait for Colleen to arrive so I could attempt to cough, she would see how pathetic it was and we would share a good laugh together, even as painful as that would be. It seemed like a great plan to me but guess who didn't bring her sense of humor that day; go figure! Oh well, like I always say, "Keep it light!"

Nh - Nutrition
80CB

Nutrition is very vital to keeping your body balanced during and after treatment. Go to your local health food store and they can assist you with the proper vitamins and herbs that help keep a sound mind and body along with helping with side effects of any medications during and after treatment. Make sure you check with your doctor before taking any herbs that may contain ingredients that might not be beneficial due to your type of cancer, such as estrogen.

One side effect of chemotherapy may be a change in your taste buds so make sure you let your doctor know if you are having trouble eating or drinking. You may have to change a few of the foods you liked until your treatment is over. Many cancer survivors have recommended using lemon drop candy or altoids to help produce saliva to keep your mouth moist and prevent mouth sores.

I have found that along with a healthy diet essential oils and massage therapy have helped me keep my body nourished. I also went for a session of bio-feedback and found out I was depleted in vitamin D and other vitamins. I now assist other newly diagnosed patients with a plan to help them through their treatment with a balance of nutrition, oils and counseling.

Along the way of this journey I am on, during the past seven years I have learned a lot about nutrition. My son was diagnosed with celiac disease and I have had to learn a whole new way of eating to remove all wheat and gluten from our diets. We have removed all breads from our home and what a difference it has made in the way that my body feels. I have added more fruits and vegetables along with water.

When looking for a vitamin, try to find one that meets your needs, not just one at your local grocery store that is generic. Since I am a hormone positive breast cancer survivor, it is recommended that we limit our use of soy because it is an estrogen and estrogen is not good for hormone positive breast cancer survivors. It is very hard to find a vitamin that does not contain soy or wheat so I am careful as to where I purchase my supplements and food products.

After my treatments were over and I was on the hormone therapy of tamoxifin, arimadex, lupron and femara, I had gained over 60 pounds and felt very uncomfortable with myself the more weight I gained. I looked back at a picture of my son and me right before I was diagnosed and was shocked, so right then and there I decided I needed to make a change. At first it was hard but once I learned that it is all about what we put into our mouths and the portion sizes I have been able to lose over 35 pounds. I still have a ways to go but as long as I keep trying I know I will succeed.

Daily Affirmation: My body deserves the best nourishment daily

Oo - One Day at a Time
୫୦୦ଓ

Take life one day at a time and count your blessings. Celebrate being you and share your gifts for God has only made one of you. Now is the time to start doing things for you. Pamper yourself with love, flowers, gifts and what is called "Me Time."

Having never taken time for myself, I now live by the motto that "I am on Patti McGee time." There will always be laundry or dishes to do, so don't fret. You can do them later after you have taken time for you. It took me some time to realize I was worth it and not to feel guilty for not attending events or gatherings.

My Journey through Cancer Treatment and Survival by: Frank Gallagher, 32 years old Michael Gallagher, 9 years old Arizona

On January 12, 1993, when I was 15-years-old, I was diagnosed with osteogenic sarcoma and also coccidioidimicodosis known as valley fever. At first I was thrown into shock, then I thought I was going to die, and then I became angry and fearful.

My life snowballed from that day forward. I was immediately admitted to Phoenix Children's Hospital, in Phoenix, Arizona. Because the spot in my lung was not

76

known as cancer metastasis, a cyst, or tumor, I was
scheduled for a lung biopsy and partial lung removal, and
knee biopsy and lump removal at the same time. Also at this
time I underwent MRI, bone scan, blood testing, etc.

I was so overwhelmed; I had to learn to take one day at
a time. I prayed a lot and went to counseling. It became a
lonely time for my mom and me. As predicted by doctors,
family and friends often disappear. They fear death and
don't know what to say.

Because of the type of cancer I had, my chemotherapy
was to run 72 hours slow drip for two weekends and a five
day drip the third week. Because of my weakened
condition, I usually ended up in the hospital for five to nine
days due to complications. My resting week I usually ended
up being re-admitted for transfusions and total parenteral
nutrition feedings. This was the plan for the next ten
months of my life.

I endured 19 surgeries in a 17 month period of time
trying to save my leg. I ultimately lost my left leg above the
knee three weeks before my 17th birthday and had three
modified amputations thereafter. Chemo was stopped after
six months due to kidney failure and cardiomyopathy. I
thought at that time it was a death sentence.

One of the happiest times during my ordeal, because my
prognosis was so uncertain due to treating two life
threatening diseases, was when I became a wish kid. The
Make-a-Wish Foundation gave me a fairy tale 16th birthday.
They gave my mom $250 to take my two brothers and
sisters-in-law, mom and me to Red Lobster for lunch,

stating mom was to keep me out of our apartment for two hours. When we returned we were astonished to find our apartment transformed into a teenage fairy land. There were balloons and streamers of every color imaginable covering the living room ceiling, teenage posters of a juke box, dancers and musical notes hanging all over. My bedroom floor was covered with green balloons (since my birthday is three days before St. Patrick's Day) and a top of the line JVC stereo system (my wish because I knew it would last a long time as opposed to a trip) was set up with a $250 gift certificate to buy CDs, tapes, etc. We were so awed we all cried, almost missing the huge birthday cake with sparklers. This was truly life inspiring for me at the lowest time of my life.

During my chemo treatment I lost every piece of hair on my body, except for some strange reason not my mustache. My oncologist would tease me constantly saying she was going to get it eventually. It never happened to her bafflement, so on my last visit to her I shaved it off.

My life was changed during this period by learning to accept what life throws at you. Don't give up. And adapt to what is, let go of what was and move forward. Take baby steps if necessary. And pray often, for there truly is power in prayer.

While I was still dealing with the aftereffects from my chemo-ravished body, my 5-month-old nephew was diagnosed with being born with a very rare form of lung cancer (pleuropulmanary blastoma). There were only 60 known cases on the books and no known cases of an infant. Luckily, a doctor at St. Jude's Hospital had treated two toddlers and was able to advise his oncologist to some degree. I am happy to say he just celebrated his 9th birthday.

While we feel so blessed to have two children survive cancer, it is sad to say there are no agencies out there who offer any financial help. My sister-in-law, who was making $45,000 a year, had to quit her job to care for her son, unable to work for over a year. Because of this and a lousy insurance plan, it cost $500 a month for the baby's chemo treatments. It took approximately 5 years for the snowball effect to catch up, but ultimately my brother and his family lost their home, cars, and had no choice but to file bankruptcy. It seems so unfair that you not only have to endure so much pain in your struggle to live, but also have to endure financial disaster, but as my sister-in-law says, we now have a healthy son. Things can always be replaced in time, and we are just starting from scratch.

If I met someone just diagnosed with cancer, I would share my 17-year survival story and tell them don't give up. A year of hell and no hair are worth more years of life cancer free.

Remember you first and happiness comes from the inside.

Pp - Patience and Perseverance
∞∞

Throughout your journey you are going to have to be patient with your progress and also persevere at trying times. It takes time to heal from surgery, chemotherapy treatments and other treatments. Your body will need to recover from fatigue and changes due to the medicines. Remember to keep a positive attitude and if you feel you are not progressing the way you feel you should, seek medical counseling. Sometimes just talking to someone can help your progress.

Perseverance
By Lisa Billington
Oneida, NY

PERSEVERANCE ... is what it takes to beat cancer. Perseverance is strength, determination, hope and faith.

When I was 15-years-old I was a diagnosed with non hodgkin's lymphoma bone cancer. I was an active young soccer player who was enjoying high school when I began having pain in my right knee. I was back and forth to many different doctors and then I was sent to a children's hospital in Pennsylvania. There, I underwent many tests, scans and a biopsy. I traveled back to Syracuse with a diagnosis of osteomyelitis, but my doctor didn't agree with the hospital's diagnosis. My doctor persevered in his search for the truth and referred me to an oncologist. The following week the oncologist sent me on a plane to St. Jude's Children's Hospital in Memphis, Tennessee. It was my first plane ride.

St. Jude's is a children's hospital that was founded by
actor Danny Thomas. St. Jude's treats thousands of
children with cancer regardless of a family's ability to pay.
This was wonderful, because at this time my father had lost
his job and money was tight. Although a hospital, St. Jude's
is a place of love and faith. Their doctors and scientists
work diligently to help cure this horrible disease. I stayed at
St. Jude's Hospital for one week and it was the most difficult
week of my life. They told my parents and me that there
were no guarantees and if I did survive I would most likely
never be able to have children of my own due to the severe
drugs I would need to take. During my stay, I went through
another needle biopsy, a spinal tap and numerous scans and
x-rays. It was there they diagnosed me with cancer and I
underwent my first round of chemotherapy. The drugs
were very strong and back in 1983 there were no drugs to
curb the nausea, so I was violently sick. I would throw up
sometimes five to ten times per hour. It was exhausting and
draining. After my first treatment, I was sent back home to
Syracuse where I was admitted to the hospital because I
was so weak and dehydrated. I continued with eight
months of chemotherapy and radiation treatments. One of
the worst parts of the treatments was that my hair fell out.
Being 15 and walking around school with hats and scarves
was not ideal, but my school and my friends were of great
support to me at that time. I also had just started dating a
boy who did not care if my hair fell out; he actually helped
me pull it out when it started falling out all over the place.
He was there through everything, the treatments, the
hospital stays, the tearful moments sitting in the car when I
did not want to burden my parents, and the Friday nights
when I had to stay home from the school sporting events

because my blood counts were low. He was an angel. Eight years later, I married him and we have been married for 18 years and we have two children.

It was a very difficult time because my friends tried to understand, but no one really knew what I was experiencing. I would lie in bed at night and wonder if I was going to die and I would wonder who would come to my funeral. It was during these dark days that I turned to my faith in God. As a child I grew up in a Catholic home and attended church on Sundays, but it was through the carrying of this cross that my faith grew. When you have nothing left but faith, you give all of your struggles to Him and pray for strength to help you persevere in your fight. You have to believe that you will get better; you have to fight to beat it, and you have to be determined to never give up. It's OK to get mad. It's OK to be sad. You will have good days and bad ones too, but you need to have hope.

Looking back, so much good did come from this terrifying experience. I know I have an amazing group of friends and unique bond with my family. I have also had many people who unfortunately have had similar battles with cancer and I know it is helpful to share my story with them, letting them know they are not alone. As strange as it seems, getting cancer was a gift in many ways because it taught me how to help others, how to pray and how to appreciate every day.

"Faith pulls us from the shadows
and sets us in the light"
- Julie Hanna, (2007 Lessons for Life Calendar)

Qq - Question, Question, Question
८०೮₃

Whether you are at a doctor's appointment, picking up a prescription or having a test done do not be afraid to ask questions about your treatment, medications or the test. Remember knowledge is power to help you through your treatment and journey. There is no such thing as a stupid question and always keep the information slips that come with your prescriptions. They list a lot of the side effects. Your doctor should also be able to give you information on the treatment or medication. Remember just because another patient had side effects does not always mean that you will.

I always keep the information that comes with my prescriptions in the medicine cabinet so if I have to call the doctor I have the information right there. I discard it when I refill my prescription with the new one in case there have been changes in the information. Once I called my gynecologist because I was having some side effects and she told me she couldn't believe I had the information right with me because most people throw them away. I have always been my best advocate.

Questions to ask:

✓ What are the side effects of the treatment or medications?
✓ Can I take other medications during the treatment or with other medications I am taking?
✓ Is this the best or most aggressive type of treatment for me? (Go with the BIG GUNS first)

Questions to ask: (Cont.)

✓ Is there a clinical trial available I can participate in?
✓ If I were your loved one would this be the treatment you would give them?
✓ Can the treatments cure me?
✓ What do you want me to do?
✓ What are the treatment options and who is on the leading edge of these options?
✓ How long can I wait before treating?
✓ What can I expect between now and then?

We can only grow and learn by asking.

Fighting through Adversity
By Diane Mitchelson
Fulton, NY

I was sitting in the shoe store waiting for my husband when I turned my head to look out the window. I felt something hurt in my neck and when I touched there I could feel a lump. I mentioned it at my next appointment and my endocrinologist told me it was a thyroid nodule and very common. She said not to worry about it. At subsequent appointments, I would always mention how it hurt and it was so large now you could see it bulging out of my neck. I told her I was worried about it and she said "I would worry more about my Thanksgiving dinner than the nodule ... it is nothing." This went on for three years until she finally decided to send me for an ultrasound. The radiologist recommended a fine needle biopsy and I went immediately for the procedure. I was now extremely worried and the wait for the results seemed interminable. When the biopsy came back positive for cancer I was filled with every emotion imaginable.

I was in shock of course and very scared but so angry too. I felt partly responsible for not being more assertive with the doctor but I had looked to her for reassurance and her expertise as a specialist. So much time had lapsed that the tumor had now spread outside the thyroid gland, another issue I blamed on the doctor.

The thyroid surgery wasn't as painful as past abdominal surgeries I had experienced for Crohn's disease, an intestinal autoimmune disease I have lived with most of my life. But the surgery was very intricate, involving vocal cords and major veins and arteries. I also had to have radiation to kill any remaining thyroid cells in the body.

I was recovering well until the 10th day when I started hemorrhaging rectally. I had no pain, no warning whatsoever until it happened. I became very dizzy and faint losing extreme amounts of blood. I had to have transfusions while the doctors tried in vain to find the source of bleeding. They all concurred that it had nothing to do with the thyroid surgery and decided it had to be related to the Crohn's disease. Thankfully the bleeding eventually stopped on its own only to start again one month later. Eventually I did wind up having another abdominal surgery for two separate resections. They removed the diseased intestines which caused strictures so food could not pass through. The severe inflammation can cause the bleeding.

Through this experience I learned many things. I have learned to be more assertive and speak up for myself. I do not take the doctor's word as gospel anymore and am not afraid to challenge their authority. I am not content to hear the words "don't worry about it." If I feel I need a test, I will ask for it. I have worked hard to establish a rapport with my doctors and to be a participant in my own health care. I also learned that I was much stronger mentally and physically and that I could handle adversity as well as the average person. I have made wonderful, caring friends through this experience and their support and love have guided me on my journey.

Rr - Resources
ɮ০ডঙ

There are many great resources available to help you through your journey. Seek out support groups and organizations that can help you with any concerns or questions. Get involved in events that support your cause. Start your own group if you can't find one locally that can help you.

I found it very helpful to reach out to others and to work with different groups to help me through any problems that occurred during my treatment and after. In the back of this book is a list of resources people have recommended that helped them.

If you are using the Internet please be careful which sites you use. Use only credited websites such as the American Cancer Society, Susan Komen and WebMD. In the resource section I list the top five websites recommended by the magazine "Women and Cancer" (Women and Cancer Winter 2006).

There are also free magazines you can send away for that are of great value. "Women and Cancer" and "Cure" are a couple you can order.

By reaching out to others and utilizing the resources available to you, you will grow stronger every day. If you are unsure about what an article is trying to say talk to your healthcare provider about it.

A Proactive Approach
Shelly Relyea
Oneida, NY

In May of 2006 I had a swollen lymph node behind my ear and went to the doctor to see what we should do. The doctor suggested we remove and biopsy it, and thankfully it came back benign. I was happy and went on with my life. A couple of years later in April of 2008, I noticed a hard lump in my cheek, so I went to the dentist to see if I had an infection. My dentist referred me to my regular doctor for his opinion. My doctor suggested having a surgeon take a look at the lump and the surgeon sent me to an ears nose and throat specialist. At this time I was getting very nervous because I was being referred to so many specialists and it took four months to make a decision on what to do. At the end of July, I finally had a needle biopsy. I was in a hospital room next to my stepdad who was in his last days with leukemia and lymphoma. My stepdad passed away the beginning of August and the day of his funeral I was diagnosed with follicular lymphoma. How ironic that I would be diagnosed with the same cancer as my stepdad even though we were not related. It was hard for me and my girls.

Knowing what my stepdad went through and watching him pass away, I felt like my world had stopped. I was wondering how everyone could continue living and laughing. My bone marrow has tested positive and I am considered stage four but since my symptoms are not bad I have not had to go through any treatment yet. I feel this is an advantage for me, because I have time to research new treatments and stay on top of the diagnosis. I am scared of having treatments but know that when I do, I will have my daughters by my side telling me what a strong person that I am.

I have already started being proactive by attending our local support groups, networking on Facebook and joining the Leukemia and Lymphoma Society website at LLS.org. I am fortunate to have a co-worker in the lab at Oneida Healthcare Center where I work who encourages me when I am nervous and listens to me when I need to talk.

I have learned from my doctors, reading and other resources that this is not a death sentence. I truly believe that God will only give me what I can endure so I am ready to fight for my future and make the best of it.

If I can leave you with any advice, I say learn to relax, let yourself feel and cry, but laugh lots and have fun.

Ss - Support

ೞೞಐ

Several times throughout this book I suggest seeking out
support. Support was very instrumental in helping me
through my journey. After I finished chemotherapy and
radiation, I had the fear that most cancer survivors go
through, "Am I really okay," along with many negative side
effects of medications, so still to this day I am always
seeking support. As mentioned earlier, I helped start our
local monthly support group and we hold it at our local
hospital. They are very supportive and provide us with a
nice dinner each month. I also sought out people to talk to.
I used hospice to help me move on from the loss of losing a
body part. Most people think hospice is only for individuals
who are dying, but they also help you if you have had a
mastectomy or lumpectomy or other surgery.

As my progress changed I sought out counselors and
psychotherapists to talk to. They provided me with an
outlet to discuss things that were bothering me when I
didn't want to bother my family and friends.

I have been blessed to be able to facilitate two support
groups and reach out to other survivors and patients and
help them through their journey by bringing in speakers to
talk about areas of interest to them. Our cancer support
group is not geared towards one cancer but to all cancers
so we have a diverse group.

A Coping Strategy
Linda Smith
Oneida, NY

Over 30 years ago, I was diagnosed with breast cancer and everything was going well until three years later when it metastasized to my left lung. I had to have a thorax lobectomy followed by a year of chemotherapy. With the help and support of my family I was able to work nearly every day. I would have to have chemotherapy every other Friday and would leave my office at 3:00 p.m. and drive to Syracuse for treatment. As I would leave the doctor's office, I would start crying. I believe at first I would cry because I felt sorry for myself. Then I became angry with the whole situation. I thought I had a lot of things they could take off and out of my body but I was not going to let the cancer get the best of me. I felt if I could go deep inside me and let the storm rage around, when it was over I would be all right. It was recommended that I read a book by Dr. Bernie Siegel called "Love, Medicine and Miracles" and it was a godsend for me. I learned many coping techniques from the book and among them was visualization, so each night I would visualize little rabbits going through my body searching for any cancer cells that were left. In this way, I felt I had some control over the cancer.

If you have a friend or relative with cancer, do not be nervous about calling or visiting them, just say "Hi, how are you doing today?" and they will take it from there. I believe they have a need to talk about it. I know I did.

Tt - Time
෩෬

The healing process from a cancer diagnosis and treatment takes time. Depending on your treatment it can take a while for your body to recover from your treatment and to mentally accept your diagnosis.

The saying "Time heals all wounds" applies to a cancer diagnosis. You can go through several phases of healing and acceptance. Many newly diagnosed patients go through stages of "Why me," "Am I going to die," and "Am I really okay." Some people make it through treatment with little or no problems but then when they are finished and have to wait three to six months before they see their doctor again, they worry about every little ache or pain and wonder if the cancer has returned. I can reassure you that as time goes on it gets easier and you worry less. Most doctors set you up so they see you at three month intervals, then progress to six months, and then yearly.

Why Me?
Judy Hooper
Canastota, NY

I am a ten year breast cancer survivor and am very thankful for my now cancer-free life. I was diagnosed with breast cancer in February 2000 and had a mastectomy with breast reconstruction on April 1 (no joke). Then after the pathology report showed lymph node involvement, I had a node dissection surgery on May 1. Thankfully, my nodes were clear of cancer. I resumed my life, went back to work at my job at Carrier… but life was very different for me. I looked at life through different eyes and made life changing decisions. I felt so very thankful for being spared my life and felt a strong desire to pay back. Being president of The Carrier Women's Club I started a knitting group and collected several knitted hats for women undergoing chemotherapy. Again I was thankful as I never needed chemotherapy or radiation therapy. I had stage two breast reconstruction surgery in October 2000. When I returned to my job for the second time I suddenly realized I was no longer happy working a full time job and quit my job at Carrier on January 1, 2001. My loving, caring husband came out of his retirement and took a part-time job. Life was good for me. I now had more time for my family and took care of my 92-year-old mother and three-year-old granddaughter so my daughter could work.

I was thoroughly enjoying my new life and very thankful for each new day. I didn't think I took every day for granted before my cancer diagnosis until I realized what could have happened to my life. I specifically remember one spring morning when my granddaughter and I were ready to go outside. As I walked outside hand in hand with my granddaughter on this beautiful sunny day, a special feeling came over me … I AM ALIVE … I could have died, but I didn't. God has spared me for a reason and since that day I try not to take life for granted and live everyday to its fullest. I began volunteering with the Susan Komen Breast Cancer Foundation, the American Cancer Society and Camp Good Days and Special Times.

In February 2001, I went for my routine mammogram to be given the diagnosis of breast cancer once again … no, not a recurrence, but breast cancer in my other breast. The comment to my surgeon was, "Okay, I know what to expect so please let's schedule the surgeries as soon as possible." Again, I was thankful as my sentinel node biopsy revealed no cancer in my nodes. On April 15 I had mastectomy number two with reconstruction by the same doctors I had complete trust in. I recovered well and enjoyed my life and everything in it … my family, my volunteer work, my garden. In September, I had stage two breast reconstruction and recovered well again. Life was good.

In 2003 our youngest daughter and family were living in England and I traveled to England to visit with them and bond with my three-year-old grandson. My English born son-in-law was my tour guide and took me to Scotland where I found my Scottish roots, being born in Nova Scotia. I found my family clan and the tartan that goes with my clan.

In March 2003, I was chosen by the American Cancer Society to be given the Fighting Spirit Award to be presented to me at The Coaches vs. Cancer Ball at the Turning Stone Casino. That was such a wonderful honor and it took me a while to accept "why me"… I am just living my life everyday but always being aware of treating each day as a gift and being as kind to everyone and everything in it and being strong. It was wonderful and I will never forget the special honor given me.

Life was going well until October 2003 when our 33-year-old daughter was diagnosed with breast cancer. That was very hard for me to accept. I always feared breast cancer in her lifetime … but not at such a young age. It was recommended she have genetic testing. The results were negative, but our surgeon explained that only means there are no identified mutations to date.

After much testing and consultation, our daughter had bilateral mastectomies in February 2004. Again, thankfully, due to early detection there was no cancer in her nodes and she recovered well. I was very happy to be a support to her and offer my experience to her.

In August 2004 during a routine colonoscopy and sigmoidoscopy, a polyp was found that couldn't be removed easily so on October 12 I had a colon resection. Again the pathology report was "clean." Again, I'm very thankful.

I have been cancer free and surgery-free (as well as my daughter) and am VERY thankful for each new day. I definitely do not take life for granted but live it to its fullest. I work a part-time job at St. Joseph's Hospital and feel I am where I should be…all my surgeries were at St. Joseph's and I have a good sense of paying back for all that they gave me. I also work very hard with the Carol Baldwin Breast Cancer Research Foundation as I believe research is where that cure will be found. Carol Baldwin always says; "Together we will find a cure." This research is extremely important to me in the life of my 11-year-old granddaughter, and my 39-year-old daughter as well as every woman.

I would like to recognize that during all my hospitalizations at St. Joseph's Hospital, Reverend Chris Kinnell was a much welcomed visitor to my bedside.

Yes, life is very special to me and I have the answer to my question of "Why me?" I feel I have been spared many times from death to be a very active fighter in this dreaded disease and to do whatever I can for my breast cancer "sisters."

Early detection is extremely important in the fight against cancer.

✓ Women: Please keep your mammograms, pap smears, and colonoscopies up to date.

✓ Men: Please keep your colonoscopies and PSA tests up to date.

Remember Time is Precious. Enjoy Life.

Clu - Understanding
୫ଠଓଓ

Understanding your diagnosis, treatment and post treatment options is one of the most important aspects of your journey. Make sure you always take someone with you to your appointments for a "second set of ears."

We sometimes shut down once we hear those three little words "You have Cancer" and we don't hear what else the doctor is saying. We also want to hear things in a different text than what the doctor said so that we think things aren't as bad as they may be. By having someone with you, they can help you by writing down what the doctor said and help you to discuss it with family and friends.

Three Different Stages
By Patti McGee
Oneida, NY

I remember I had researched all the information on my diagnosis that the oncologist and surgeon had given me. My sister Kelly, who was my "second set of ears," had ordered me a breast cancer guide from the American Cancer Society and as I was looking up my staging of cancer I had myself at stage two. I had a 2.5 cm tumor with one lymph node involved and no metastasis which gave me an 80% survival rate which was refreshing to me. I had just finished chemotherapy and had set up my consultation for radiation. I had always taken someone to my appointments and treatments but since it was radiation and I felt the worst was behind me, I went to the appointment alone. I had dropped my son off at his Aunt Sandy's and told her I would be back soon. During my consultation, the radiotherapist was going over the procedure and how long I would have to have radiation and then he said, "Since you are stage three aggressive" and at that point I felt nauseous and wanted to cry. He must have sensed it and said, "No one told you your cancer is aggressive." I said "No I am stage two." At that point nothing else mattered because in all my research, I remember that if I was stage three aggressive that my rate of survival dropped to around 50% from 80%. I couldn't wait to get out of his office and call my surgeon who had given me my tumor size and lymph nodes involved.

As I left the office, everything was going through my mind again. Did I make the right decision on a lumpectomy versus a mastectomy? Was I going to live to see my son grow up, he was 9-years-old at that time, and everything was running through my mind. I picked my son up and his aunt calmed me down and I called my surgeon. It seemed like days but he finally called me back and he agreed that it was stage three but not aggressive, so I felt a little better but now I had three different stages. How could that be? I had my first recheck with my oncologist, within a few weeks, so I waited to talk to her. I trusted her and the oncology office with my life and knew she had planned my treatment around the diagnosis. I met with Dr. Lemke and she went over the tumor size and lymph nodes involved and we agreed on stage two. It was a huge relief and to this day I have felt comfortable with the decision. I truly believe that if it was stage three aggressive, it would have been recommended that I have a mastectomy.

As I was going through treatment and post treatment I had some difficult times from nausea, vomiting, double eye infections, chest infection and other side effects. I have learned not to just accept all suggestions from my doctors but to research and understand why they want me take a medication or have a treatment and what the side effects are. I have a much better understanding of my body and how it works than I have ever had and treat it like it is fragile. I exercise, have changed my eating habits, have sought out the use of essential oils and receive massages regularly. I have learned to slow down, to tell people "no" if I do not want to do something and not feel guilty because I have let them down, and I have learned to live life for me.

Cancer had changed my life so much for the better that I left my job of 17 ½ years to become a massage therapist and now I reach out to others through mind, body and spirit to help them through their journey. It was one of the best decisions I could have ever made in my life. I am the happiest I have ever been.

Be your own advocate, because only you know your body and how you are feeling.

V - Value

ℬᴑᴄᴊ

If you didn't value your health prior to your diagnosis now is the time to get in tune with your body because only you know when something doesn't feel right. Do not be afraid to seek second opinions or to change doctors if you do not feel comfortable with your current physician. Seek out the best possible care for you, physically, mentally and medically. I recommend you work with your doctors and set up a treatment plan for the mind and body while you are going through your treatment.

Love and Big Hugs
Jan Compoli
Oneida, NY

On Wednesday, April 7, 2004, at 4:30 pm, I had an appointment at the Oneida Surgical Group for the results of my breast biopsy. As I sat there in the reception area, I realized that I was going to be the last patient of the day. I thought that was a bit odd, but thought nothing more of it. My name was finally called and I went into the examination room. My surgeon came into the room and said, "Jan you have a melanoma." I just sat there staring at him thinking, "What did he say? Was he talking to me? Was there someone else in the room?" My surgeon then said, "Jan, did you hear me? I said you have cancer." I just nodded my head, kind of numb. Actually I was thinking "OH SHIT!" How could this be? There was no history of cancer in my family. My doctor asked me if my husband was with me and where we could sit and talk; he would explain to me what I was dealing with and what was next. As I sat listening to him, I could not really comprehend what he was telling me. There was too much to consume and I had not gotten over the words "Jan, you have cancer."

The next day, I had to inform my boss that I had cancer and surgery was necessary. His comment to me was, "Jan, we must schedule this around the office; we have to plan this out." I could not believe my ears. I said, "No I am sorry Dr. G. My surgery is scheduled and I will be there on Monday, April 12." I knew then that this was not going to be easy. With everything else, I now must deal with a very unreasonable boss.

I was referred for a second opinion at the Oneida oncology. My surgeon was going to schedule me for the first available appointment, because he did not want me to wait. I was scheduled for a bone scan and blood work at Oneida Healthcare Center on Friday, April 9, 2004 at 11:00 am. Another appointment was scheduled with an oncologist (Dr. M) at Oneida Oncology Group on Monday, April 12, 2004 at 1:00 pm. At my first appointment with my oncologist, I felt a little uncomfortable with him; however, I thought it must be me with all I was dealing with. Dr. M. suggested I follow my surgeon's direction and schedule for surgery. A mastectomy was too aggressive, a lumpectomy would be sufficient. So I called my surgeon's office and scheduled surgery. My pretesting was scheduled for Friday, May 7, at OHC at 9:30 am. My surgery was scheduled for Monday, May 10 at 11:30 am and I needed to be at OHC at 8:30 am.

My follow-up appointment for lab results was scheduled on Monday, May 17 at 9:15 am. Results: I did not have clear margins; we needed to schedule more surgery ASAP. I was scheduled for Wednesday, May 19, at 7:45 am, at OHC at 6:00 am. In the meantime, I had another appointment with Dr. M, my oncologist on Monday, May 14 at 8:30 am. I was beginning to realize that I am very uncomfortable with this person and when finished with my appointment, I sat in my car and cried.

My follow-up appointment after surgery was scheduled with my surgeon on Wednesday, May 26, at 4:15 pm. I was informed that I finally had clear margins and that my next step would be radiation.

On Monday, June 2, I had another appointment with Dr. M. and again I left unhappy. We are not on the same page. He said I must change my attitude; what is wrong with me? I must be trying too hard to deal with everything. My boss is giving me a hard time about leaving work for so many appointments, and my oncologist tells me I must change my attitude toward my boss and understand what my boss must be going through without me. Are you kidding me? I just don't believe this guy.

Wednesday, June 9, at 3:00 pm I see Dr. D. at Oneida Radiology. WOW, I love this woman. She is wonderful. She takes her time talking with me and explaining what will be happening. Appointments are scheduled for mapping, tattooing, and radiation appointments which will be every day for eight weeks. Next appointment will be June 24 to begin process of radiation.

I have appointments every day at 3:30 pm for radiation; these appointments do not set well with my boss. He gives me a hard time every single day when I have to leave. I have had to tell my boss that my appointments are at 3:00 because I know he will keep me as late as he can and will make me late. I cannot afford to miss any of my radiation appointments. This is very stressful.

In the meantime, I have follow-up appointments with my surgeon, and my oncologist. Every day I am dealing with my boss asking me, "How much longer is this going to go on Jan?" I said, "Well Dr. G., not much longer."

Now, my husband has gone for a stress test and it is decided that he must go for a catherization because something showed up in his stress test. Appointments are now scheduled for my husband. I must have my radiation daily. This will be tricky. Everything works out because my radiologist will meet me very early in the morning before my husband's surgery so I will not miss an appointment. They are just wonderful. Then we are off to Utica and St. Elizabeth's for my husband. Stents are necessary and surgery is scheduled for my husband. It all worked out and my husband is doing well.

On August 20, 2004, I receive my certificate for completing radiation. Oh my goodness, I have finally completed everything. I cannot believe it. I cry like a baby, realizing what I have been through and I made it. I am continuing to see my oncologist and still not happy with him. He does not make me feel good about myself.

One thing I have done for myself was to give my two week notice at work. I have had enough of this Dr. G. I cannot believe how much better I feel. I probably shouldn't have, but I told him exactly what I thought of him. OK, Jan, this is for you. Chin up, kiddo, you are a good person and no one will ever treat you poorly again.

November 5, 2004, I have an appointment with my surgeon; he tells me I have an infection and places me on medication. December 27, 2004 I have my first mammogram after surgery. The mammogram shows that I have an infection; the picture is very cloudy, and they are concerned. An appointment is scheduled for me so I went to my surgeon for more medication to try to clear it up. After a few months, the infection is still there and surgery will be necessary. The problem is I have an inverted nipple which is moist all the time causing the infection. This must be removed. Oh my God, I really cannot believe this. Will this ever end? I am referred to another surgeon for removal of this and realize this is the hardest of all surgeries. I will be awake while they are cutting off my nipple. OK, I have handled everything else, I will get through this. This surgery is scheduled for April 5, 2005. It has been almost one year since my diagnosis and since I began this process.

In the meantime, on Wednesday, February 2, a support group had been started in the Oneida Area. I decide that I must go and see what this is all about. I definitely need some support. I am not handling all this very well. I need some advice on what to do about my oncologist. I cannot continue to see this oncologist any longer. I need someone who will help me feel better about myself. The support given to me at this support group was awesome. This is a great group of very supportive people. I was advised to take charge of my treatment and inform my doctors I was unhappy and uncomfortable with my oncologist. I spoke with my surgeon and he suggested I call the Oneida oncology office to see what steps I needed to take to make a change in my doctors. I had to call Dr. M. and tell him I was uncomfortable having him as my doctor and that I would be more comfortable seeing a woman doctor. I was asked who I would like to see and the transfer was made. I am now so very happy with my oncologist. She is wonderful and I have thanked her for taking me as her patient. We must be our own advocate and if we are unhappy or uncomfortable seeing anyone, speak up and make the necessary changes. It was harder thinking and worrying about it than actually doing it.

After my April 5, 2005 surgery and the removal of my nipple is when I start to spiral downward. I cannot handle this anymore. OK God, please get me through this, one day at a time.

May 4, 2005, I saw my oncologist and was placed on an antidepressant medication. I am crying all of the time. Feel like I am just not able to pull myself together. After all this, now I am depressed. Why? I am usually a happy person able to handle anything. Now I am unable to get out of bed without crying. I take my shower and cry, cry, cry.

After taking the medication for a couple of weeks, I do start to feel better. The dots are beginning to reconnect. Time really does heal. My journey has been difficult, but I am a survivor. At an I Can Cope Series in Oneida, a wonderful woman from Faxton Breast Care Center discussed partial prosthetics that are available for women. I scheduled an appointment with her and I have a new prosthesis and bra to wear and I am now comfortable with my body and how I look. Watch out world, here comes Jan. I cannot believe that I was not aware of this sooner. After 5 ½ years of wearing jackets to cover myself up because I was embarrassed at how I look, now I am feeling better and able to get on with my life. I have recently retired and life could not be better. I am now a six year survivor. I thank God every day for such a wonderful life.

One thing I keep telling others is to try to take one day at a time; the big picture is too overwhelming. Just take it one small step at a time. You can make it. I did.

The question is not "why me," but, "why not me?" I would not wish this on anyone else. Go to support group, because you will meet some wonderful people and every one of us has a story to tell. Each journey is a little different, but worth hearing.   I have made many prayer shawls for cancer patients and feel good about giving back when I can. My best friends are cancer survivors. They know what it is like and how to live. It has been very difficult for me to tell my story. I just feel I must get on with living. Now that I have written it down, I am glad that I did. I hope my story will help someone.

W W – Water, Water, Water
ᏉᏟᏘ

Water is one of our most vital resources. The body is made up of approximately 98% water and during treatment you are going to have to increase your intake to stay hydrated. The medicines used can dehydrate you and if you have side effects of vomiting or diarrhea you will have to stay hydrated. It can be tough at times to drink enough water but if you carry a bottle with you at all times you can sip on it throughout the day for maximum efficiency of the body. Water hydrates the joints and muscles and can alleviate body aches and pains.

In my training as a licensed massage therapist it is recommended to drink half your body weight in ounces; so for example a 150 pound individual should drink 75 ounces of water per day. If you can, try to drink more to stay hydrated. Many people think that by drinking sugary waters or flavored drinks they will keep you hydrated but the best most effective way is pure water. If you don't like the taste of plain water try adding fresh lemons or other fruit to your glass or bottle.

It is recommended to drink water at room temperature to avoid constriction of your blood vessels. If you must drink ice cold water, try to balance your system with a warm drink, such as a green tea with antioxidants. Water flushes toxins out of your body.

As your treatments continue, your body will build up toxins from the drugs that are used to treat your cancer. Through the use of Epsom salts you can detoxify your body by soaking in bath water and one cup of Epsom salts. If you prefer you can add essential oils to the bath water to sooth aches and pains, boost your immune system and relax you from the stresses of your diagnosis. Please discuss any complementary treatments with your healthcare provider to make sure it will not interfere with treatment. Your local health store can recommend oils and vitamins or minerals. Do your research and seek out knowledgeable holistic healers to assist in your treatment.

Drink your Water and Fight
Deb Debiase
Oneida, NY

My name is Deborah D. and I am a six year survivor. I was diagnosed on September 11, 2003 with Non-Hodgkin B-Follicular Lymphoma. (Stage III). It all started with one little lump. Then, before I knew it, I was sitting in a room with fellow survivors, an IV in my arm, wondering how this could have happened to me. Looking around I soon realized that if these people can do this, well then, so can I.

After the initial shock of it all I proceeded to see myself as not having the dreaded "Big C" ... Cancer. I was simply sick and would do what I have to get back on track again. So every three weeks I sat with an IV in my arm, drinking my never ending mega cup of water, chatting with my fellow survivors. Before chemotherapy I was not a big fan of the life sustaining liquid called water. But to this day I am forever drinking it. Through chemotherapy I knew that this was the one way to help my body rid itself of the toxins that were removing the cancer cells and in return making me feel like I was run over by a Mack truck. As these drugs were being pumped into my body, the cool refreshing water was helping to flush them out. Simply put, drinking the cold liquid (always with lots of ice) made me feel better.

Before my adventure with "C" I never really paid too much attention to the many people whose lives were affected by this dreaded disease. The many people who had their daily routine interrupted and turned upside down. Now as I look around, there are so many that have ridden and are on the "C" ride.

When I have the privilege to meet someone who has to ride that roller coaster I have these words of wisdom that I tell them.

1. This diagnosis is by no means a death sentence.

2. It is by no means fun. As the saying goes "Cancer Sucks."

3. This is something you can deal with, fight and conquer.   And somehow we do.

This ride has changed me as I am sure it does for everyone. I now enjoy my birthdays as they signify yet another year I have dealt with, fought and conquered and in short survived. I truly believe that every day is a gift and to live life to the fullest. One never knows what is lurking around the corner.

So go through the endless CT Scans, blood work, PET scans, and chemo. Drink your water and fight.

YOU CAN DO THIS!

Xx - X-rays
ಬಂಡ

X-rays are going to become part of your life so ask your doctors to show you how to read them. You will feel much better after you have reviewed them personally and can understand what the doctor is seeing and explaining to you.

I would recommend going to an imaging center that has a doctor on staff to tell you your results immediately. I know of so many women who go for mammograms and have to wait a week or so for the results to be mailed to them or they get all the way home and have to come back for more x-rays. Once you have had cancer you want to get the results as quickly as possible.

If you have any scars or marks on the skin area that will be x-rayed remind the technician to mark them so when they show up on the x-ray there is no question as to what it is. In 2003, I went for my first mammogram after having surgery and completing treatment; I was very nervous and scared. It was about three months after radiation and five after chemotherapy I was happy to be done with everything and I had convinced my oncologist to remove the port they put in to administer chemotherapy, which she really thought should stay in a little longer but I wanted it removed. I had a scar from the removal of the port just above my left breast and the technician did not mark it. After taking x-rays of both breasts, I was sitting in the little waiting room that they provide. It usually doesn't take that long for them to come back and tell me everything was clear, but on this particular day, I was sitting and waiting what seemed like forever and I was getting nervous and wanted to cry. I must have waited at least 15 minutes and the room felt like it was getting smaller. Finally, the technician came in and said they wanted to do an ultrasound of the left breast because they thought they saw something unusual and it concerned them. All those thoughts of recurrence and metastasis came rushing through my mind. I thought this cannot be happening; didn't the chemotherapy work? I could see the compassion in the radiologist's eyes. As we got ready to do the ultrasound, as soon as I exposed my left breast and he saw the scar he knew what was on the x-ray. We did the ultrasound anyway to rule out any abnormality but it could have all been avoided if the scar had been marked properly, so now I make sure I remind the technician to mark the scars. I left the Imaging Center with two pink carnations that day. It truly scared both the radiologist and me.

Early Detection a One in a Million Catch
Tena Roache
Oneida, NY

I had been going for mammograms for over 20 years, when in 2007 one changed my life. After reading the films the radiologist suggested I go and see a surgeon so they made an appointment for me with Dr. Kelly. I had to wait a couple weeks; I was so scared and it was the longest two weeks of my life. I finally went to the appointment and when they invite you into the conference room you know something is not right. Thankfully I brought my friend Shirley and she went in with me. Dr. Kelly gave me three choices: I could wait six months and do nothing to see if anything changes; I could take an experimental pill; or I could have a mastectomy. A big choice, right?

Dr. Kelly told me to think about it for a couple of weeks and in that time I really didn't know which decision was the best but I did know that I just wanted the cancer out of my body. The waiting was driving me crazy wondering if it was spreading. I finally decided to have a mastectomy, so on May 29, 2007 I had a double mastectomy. Dr. Kelly told me he felt he got all the cancer and there would only be a two percent chance that the cancer would return.

Dr. Kelly referred me to an oncologist, so I took my films over to the Oneida Oncology Department to Dr. Lemke. After reviewing my films and report, Dr. Lemke said that I was one in a million to catch the cancer before it spread. Since Dr. Lemke works in a teaching hospital, she asked if she could keep my films and show them to the students in her classes because the cancer cells were so small and usually go undetected. I let her keep them and hope that they will help save someone else from this disease. I was fortunate that I did not need any further treatment and have to continue to see Dr. Kelly on a yearly basis.

It is never easy when you have been told you have cancer regardless of the type of cancer or the type of treatment, but I just pray to God that it never comes back.

I encourage everyone to get screened regularly for all types of cancers and hopefully early detection can save your life.

STAY STRONG!

𝒴𝓎 - 𝒴ou
ଔଔଔ

You are the most important person throughout your journey so make yourself a priority. Rest when you feel tired, only do the things that you feel you want to do and feel comfortable doing. As time goes on you will feel more comfortable going out in public and will get stronger mentally and physically. Just because you completed your treatment doesn't mean your journey ends there. You will begin to rethink where you are in your life and you may want to make some changes. Include your family and friends in any major changes you want to make so that they feel part of the decision. They have been there for you since the beginning and will want to help you throughout the rest of your journey.

Remember to take it one day at a time. Breathe when things get stressful. Make sure you take care of yourself. Reach out to others and you will find self gratification.

Healing Your Body and Soul
Julie Baum
Utica, NY

In the fall of 2007, at the age of 43, I noticed a change in my nipple that turned out to be nothing, but saved my life. My partner casually mentioned that my nipple looked different, almost misshapen. I didn't think anything of it, but I was having a physical that week so I had my nurse practitioner check it. This began a whirlwind of doctors and treatments that seemed to last much longer than it actually did. My physical exam was normal, but my nurse practitioner suggested we do my yearly mammogram sooner than later and an appointment was scheduled for the following week. I didn't think much about it until the radiologist called the day after my mammogram and told me that they would need to do an ultrasound and a biopsy. I still didn't think much of it because I had talked to so many women who said that they had lumps and had biopsies that turned out to be nothing. Some went back year after year to have things checked that never amounted to anything. So I was a little nervous, but not worried.

I went to my biopsy appointment and was told that my concerns over my nipple were unfounded and that the change in shape was a normal part of the aging process. Great! However, when my doctor did my biopsy, he said that there was a lot of bleeding because there was a small artery going to the lump which was by now palpable. I knew right then, that if it had a blood supply, it wanted to grow and that it was probably cancer. Within a couple days I got the news that I had been diagnosed with Invasive Ductile Carcinoma. This was the scariest time for me, my partner and my family. I had another appointment in a week with the breast care doctor who did the biopsy. It was the longest week of my life. Once we came up with a game plan of lumpectomy, chemotherapy and radiation, life was better. The waiting and not knowing what the "treatment" would be was the toughest part of the whole experience for me.

My surgery was actually one of the easiest parts of my treatment for me due to the fact that I was able to keep most of my breast. Chemotherapy was a whole different story and there was nothing easy about it. I became dehydrated twice and had two trips to the Oncologist and Urgent Care to be hydrated. The day-to-day issues of trying to keep up with my job, home, family and basically life was difficult. I remember lying on my couch on my bad days when I just couldn't make it to work and looking out at the winter landscape just waiting for time to pass. I would look at the winter themed flag hanging outside of our living room window and think 'Soon the Valentines flag will go up and I will be that much closer to being done with chemo.' I knew in May we would hang the flag with the flowers on it in honor of spring and I would be done. I would envision the leaves budding on the tree and that Spring flag everyday I spent on the couch. I smiled the entire time I put that flag up and probably always will. Chemotherapy is a cumulative poisoning of your body to cure cancer and by the end, I felt pretty beat up yet triumphant.

My partner, my family, and my friends all stepped up to the plate during my treatments. People brought food, sent fun DVDs in the mail and sometimes just sat and listened when I needed to talk about what I was going through. My partner Karen would field phone calls from everyone when I didn't have the energy to talk. She would experiment with foods for me to eat during chemo and cooked any time I was hungry and felt like eating. (Soft boiled eggs and toast seemed to always stay down and felt good in my stomach!) Karen sat with me at most of my appointments and wrote in my notebook what was being discussed so we would remember everything discussed later. She held my hand and rubbed my back when I just wanted to stop the world from turning. She was awesome through the whole experience!

My family would come and sit with me at home when Karen couldn't be there and I often thought of people who lived alone and how they made it through chemo. I was lucky to have my mother, father, stepmother, sister and my partner's sister all accompany me to chemo and know firsthand what I was going through to get better. My mother gave me Dr. Susan Love's Breast Book for Christmas that year and it was my Bible throughout treatment. They were all wonderful which only reaffirmed what a great family I have.

My co-workers also pitched in to make life more bearable. I took a few days off after every chemo, but worked through my treatments, which was not easy. When I went to my job, people actually expected me to work! Fortunately, my supervisors were wonderful and provided an environment that enabled me to continue working when I was sick. My co-workers each took turns having their pictures taken with me while *they* were wearing my wig which we named 'Kate'. They would help me get my lunch when I barely had the energy to be at work at all. The people I work with would field questions from other departments and just make me feel like I was still part of the hum that is a busy office. They were fantastic...

My longtime friends came and walked in our local breast cancer walk and ordered t-shirts for our "Team Big Gal". I was shocked to find that we had 40 friends and family participate in the walk. I then realized how much I was loved. Some old friends didn't come around while I was sick for their own reasons and that was ok. Many of my acquaintances stepped up to the plate and were great. They developed into friends that I could count on to help get me through a dark time. I believe that happens with any life crisis and cancer is no exception, but I hadn't expected the outpouring of support.

For me, radiation turned out to be a simple process of just showing up every day. Compared to chemo, it was a breeze and the weeks flew by. By the time I had finished with my treatments in June 2008, I had made some wonderful new 'Breast' Friends. So many women whom I had not known before treatment were willing to share their story of recovery with me which helped me get through my own treatments. At first I thought "Don't these women just want to put it all behind them?" I didn't understand that I would want to help other women get through what I had already been through. At the time, I didn't understand that helping others through treatment would help me continue to heal my body and soul by sharing my story.

Many wonderful things happen during my cancer journey. I found my local chapter of the American Cancer Society was a great resource with caring people and great programs to assist me through my cancer journey. I had wonderful doctors, but the nurses I met, especially at chemotherapy, became like family during my treatment. They offered what we needed before we asked and took time to answer all of our questions. When one of my chemo nurses heard me whining about having to be careful when eating fresh fruits and vegetables, he threw his hands up, laughed and said "We are trying to cure cancer here, you know!" I still take in batches of chocolate chip cookies when I go in for checkups, but will never be able to show them how important they were to my recovery.

I have found that people approach cancer the same way they approach everything else in life. Having a positive attitude about life definitely makes treatments easier. I try to look at the good things in my experience and let the rest fall to the wayside. I know that it could all change at any time, but I try to enjoy each day and spend my time in ways that make me happy. Recently, Dr. Jerri Nielson Fitzgerald passed away from a recurrence of Breast Cancer. She had been at the South Pole during Polar Winter and had to deal with her diagnosis as well as her treatment via email to her doctor. At a lecture in Denver she had said "I would rather not have it. But the cancer is part of me. It's given my life color and texture." It has given *my* life "color and texture" and helps me to enjoy each day in ways that I am still learning to appreciate.

What Cancer Cannot Do

Cancer is so limited…
It cannot cripple love.
It cannot shatter hope.
It cannot corrode faith.
It cannot eat away peace.
It cannot destroy confidence.
It cannot kill friendship.
It cannot shut out memories.
It cannot silence courage.
It cannot reduce eternal life.
It cannot quench the spirit.
Anonymous

Ze - Zest
🙰🙴

You have been dealt an obstacle that you can overcome. Through laughter and faith your zest for life will shine through. Try to focus on the positives in your life: peace, love and happiness, because in the end that is all that matters. Surround yourself with positive caring people and don't be afraid to make changes in your life or your career. Your priorities may change and don't be afraid to live out your dreams. "Follow your dreams; for as you dream, so shall you become" (James Allen).

"All the wonders that you seek are within yourself"
- Sir Thomas Browne

A Sign from God
Penny Poling
Sherrill, NY

July 18, 2002 - It was a joyous occasion; my husband, Paul and I were getting ready for his daughter's wedding in Niagara Falls, Canada. I was in the shower and felt a small "lump" in my right breast. It concerned me a little bit, but my first thought was, "It feels like my rib, sort of," and pretty much dismissed it at that.

Paul was a little insistent that I be seen. We came home from the trip and I waited about a week to make the appointment but when I did call, I couldn't be seen for

about two weeks. No problem; I kept the appointment.
Well, I happened to see my OBGYN, Mickey Moore, the
very next day at Rotary and mentioned that I had made the
appointment because of the little bump (about the size of a
pea) and she said, "I will see you tomorrow morning at 9:00
a.m." She examined me and suggested I have my surgeon
take a look so she called Dr. Lindsey from her office and
insisted I be seen as soon as possible. I got into his office a
few days later. He then sent me to Oneida Imaging to have
a mammogram and ultrasound. The ultrasound clearly
showed the lump and several clusters of calcifications (pre-
cancer cells). I was set up to have the calcifications
removed in mid-August and the lump removed a week or
so after that. The procedure was basically painless. The
lumpectomy was done in the operating room as an
outpatient procedure. It obviously was sore for a few days.
It is now Labor Day Weekend and I couldn't stand not
knowing the results so I left a message with the doctor's
answering service. He called back shortly with the news,
"It's cancer." He told me to think about having a
mastectomy because I had had another lump removed in
1997 in the same breast that was considered "borderline
cancer," so in my opinion, it was the only way to get rid of
the cancer once and for all. Well, you can only imagine the
thoughts and emotions that flooded me (I thought, I am only
42 years old. I have a lifetime ahead of me with my husband
and daughter and friends). As Paul and I sat in the kitchen
digesting this horrific news, a hummingbird came to the
feeder outside the kitchen window. The window was open
halfway with a screen in it. The bird perched and drank the
sugar and water mixture. It wasn't the first time I had seen
the bird but the strange thing was that my cat jumped in the
window, and the bird just stayed there perched and
drinking. I thought, THAT IS WEIRD; hummingbirds are

pretty skittish. My next thought was it has to be a sign from God that I was going to be OK and that he was going to take care of me and get me through what lay ahead. Well, I decided that I needed that reassurance and prayed to see the sign again. I prayed to see that hummingbird back at the feeder. Well, I must have sat in the kitchen for 20 minutes at a time waiting for that stupid thing. A couple of days went by without any sighting, and then, I received a card from an old friend and former co-worker with a hummingbird in 3D. My prayers had been answered. It's funny how God answers prayers just sometimes not the way you would expect.

I had the mastectomy on September 20 (four days after my 42nd birthday). It really wasn't too painful but the scar looked horrendous (36 staples). I spent the next couple of months going to physical therapy, because when they take your lymph nodes under your arm it's difficult and painful to get your arm up and over your head. But the good news was that the nodes were negative. I then saw my oncologist, Dr. John Gullo. He was also my mother's cancer doctor. He suggested that I receive chemotherapy. I was set up for four treatments - three weeks apart. The treatments consisted of cytoxin and andreamycyin. It was pretty lethal stuff, and yes I was probably going to lose my hair. Dr. Lindsey surgically implanted a port in my chest three days before chemo on October 15 so that the toxic chemicals would not damage the veins in my arms. My first treatment started October 18, ironically my mother's birthday. The room was large with a lot of recliners. I saw people of all ages (I was the youngest) hooked up getting their various choices of cocktails. I got through it without too much trouble. Actually I felt pretty good, but by noon the next day I crashed. I was pretty nauseated for the next few days; the anti-nausea meds offered some relief. Three more to go! All with the same ill feeling and lasting about five days.

Friday, November 1, exactly two weeks after my first treatment, I was showering and all of a sudden I had hair between my fingers, running down my face, I looked down at my feet and saw one big clump of hair. How awful. I called Paul to come home from work and comfort me. I spent the next day coming to terms with my hair loss. In the evening, I decided to just shave my head. At least I was in control of losing the rest of it. I was ready for the wig (well, you're never really ready). It took a while for me to feel comfortable and not so self-conscious about it. My last treatment was December 26. My hair started to grow back in February. I remember going to the store one day and as I went to get out of the car my wig got caught on the door and came off and I remember diving back into the car to put it back on and looked around to make sure no one saw me. I remember sitting there laughing.

Well, with that over, I started thinking about breast reconstruction. Why not; I've gone this far and have been through a lot. I met with Dr. Anthony DeBoni in Syracuse, NY and scheduled surgery for July 2, 2003. It was a 6 ½ hour major surgery called a tram flap. A tram flap is where they take the fat from your stomach to make the new breast and they also have to tunnel the blood supply up under the skin and connect it to your underarm. After a year and three minor surgeries I finally "looked normal." It was all worth it.

I am celebrating seven years now and consider myself a true survivor but there is still not a day that goes by that I don't think about cancer and that nasty little word "recurrence." I just know that I did all the right things and had the best absolute care. I also know that cancer is no longer a death sentence, but just a mere hurdle, a speed bump in the road to life. Early detection is the key to survival and don't ever take anything for granted.

I have only seen the hummingbird a few times since 2002 but everywhere I am, whether it be camping or shopping and I see a hummingbird, I am reminded that God is near. I attended Camp Good Days and Special Times in Buffalo, NY and on the last day, we spent some time at an outdoor church, reflecting on the weekend. As I quietly sat and cried, someone passed me a box of tissues and the box had hummingbirds on it. Yet another little reminder that God is always near.

Resources and References

Referred Books:

Just get me through this!: The Practical Guide to Breast Cancer by Deborah A. Cohen.

For the Love of Teddy; The Story Behind Camp Good Days and Special Times by Lou Buttino

The Ph Miracle Diet: Balance Your Diet, Reclaim Your Health by Robert O. Young and Shelley Redford Young

Love, Medicine and Miracles by Dr. Bernie Siegel, MD

The Secret by Rhonda Byrne

It's Not About the Bike by Lance Armstrong

The Bible

90 Minutes in Heaven: A True Story of Death & Life by Don Piper, Cecil Murphey

The Five People You Meet in Heaven by Mitch Albom

2007 Lessons For Life Calendar by Julie Hanna and Ellen Anderson.

Recommended Free Magazines:

Cure Magazine
3102 Oak Lawn Ave, Suite 610
Dallas, Texas 75219 USA

Women & Cancer

Recommended Music:

Bad Day - Daniel Powter
Calling All Angels - Train
I Hope You Dance - Lee Ann Womack
Live like You Were Dying - Tim McGraw CD
Stronger Than Before - Olivia Newton -John CD
My Wish - Rascal Flatts
Skin - Rascal Flatts
The Road - Chad Mackey CD
The Climb - Miley Cyrus
I Will Survive - Gloria Gaynor
The Fall - Nora Jones
I Run for Life - Melissa Ethridge

Recommended Websites:

www.cancer.org - American Cancer Society
www.womenandcancermag.com - Women & Cancer
www.campgooddays.org - Camp Good Days and Special Times
www.cancerconsultants.com
www.caringbridge.org
www.cancer.gov - National Cancer Institute
www.oncolink.com
www.webmd.com
www.lls.org - Leukemia & Lymphoma Society
www.susankomen.org - Susan Komen Foundation
www.findacure.org - Carol Baldwin Breast Cancer Foundation
www.curetoday.com - Cure Magazine
www.WomensHealth@everydayhealth.com
www.stjude.org - St. Jude's Children's Hospital
www.upstate.edu - SUNY Upstate Medical University -
                        University Hospital
www.mayoclinic.com - The Mayo Clinic, Rochester, MN
www.mdanderson.org - MD Anderson, Houston, TX
www.consumermedsafety.org
www.safemedication.com

About the Author:

Patti McGee, an inspiration to many cancer survivors, resides in Central New York with her son Dylan and dog Snickers. Patti's diagnosis of breast cancer has inspired her to continue to be an advocate for other cancer survivors to help them through their journey. In 2004 she teamed up with Oncology Nurse Practitioner, Karen Litwak, to start The Oneida Area Relay For Life through the American Cancer Society. In 2010, the Oneida Area Relay For Life reached the one million dollar mark. Patti has also been instrumental in co-chairing a monthly support group and the American Cancer Society's "I Can Cope" educational series.

In 2006, Patti was selected to be an ambassador for the American Cancer Society and lobbied Congress in Washington D.C. to keep research money in the budget to continue making progress and to one day find a cure for this dreaded disease. While in D.C. Patti was able to talk with legislators about her journey and the importance of research.

Prior to her cancer diagnosis in 2002, Patti was a recreation director, but in 2007 left the recreation profession to pursue a career in massage therapy. After her partial mastectomy in 2003, scar tissue had formed around the site and was causing some discomfort so Patti sought out a massage therapist. She found the benefits so rewarding that in 2008, after completing her schooling, she opened and continues to own her massage business Time for Reflection Massage Therapy and Resource Center.

Patti's passion for advocacy has led her to be featured in several articles such as "Miss May" in the 2008 American Cancer Society's Making Strides Against Breast Cancer

About the Author: (Cont.)

calendar, the March 17, 2010 Mending Hands Article :
Meeting of the Massage Minds and participated in the 2010
Mary Kay Fashion Show in Rome, NY. Reaching out to
other survivors has helped her to thrive in her journey
through cancer.

In 2010, Patti became a board member of the Cancer
Fund "Laurie's Legacy" which assists breast cancer patients
financially throughout their treatment in the Oneida area.
Knowing firsthand how cancer can be financially devastating
to the cancer patient, she continues to research options to
assist cancer survivors financially so they can focus on their
treatments.

Patti's goal is to donate a percentage of each book sale
to a foundation to help ease the financial burden for cancer
survivors in the Central NY area. For more information
about the author or to contact her to speak at your event
e-mail Patti at pmcgee2@twcny.rr.com or visit
www.timeforreflectionmassagetherapy.com.

8425671R0

Made in the USA
Charleston, SC
08 June 2011